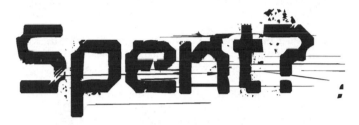

Spent?

End Exhaustion & Feel Great Again

Dr FRANK LIPMAN
with Mollie Doyle

HAY HOUSE

Australia • Canada • Hong Kong • India
South Africa • United Kingdom • United States

Published and distributed in the United Kingdom by:
Hay House UK Ltd, 292B Kensal Rd, London W10 5BE.
Tel.: (44) 20 8962 1230; Fax: (44) 20 8962 1239. www.hayhouse.co.uk

Published and distributed in Australia by:
Hay House Australia Ltd, 18/36 Ralph St, Alexandria NSW 2015.
Tel.: (61) 2 9669 4299; Fax: (61) 2 9669 4144. www.hayhouse.com.au

Published and distributed in the Republic of South Africa by:
Hay House SA (Pty), Ltd, PO Box 990, Witkoppen 2068. Tel./Fax: (27) 11 467
8904.www.hayhouse.co.za

Published and distributed in India by:
Hay House Publishers India, Muskaan Complex, Plot No.3, B-2, Vasant Kunj,
New Delhi– 110 070. Tel.: (91) 11 4176 1620; Fax: (91) 11 4176 1630. www.
hayhouse.co.in

A catalogue record for this book is available from the British Library.

Photography by Beth Galton
Designed by Mary Austin Speaker

Published in the United States of America by Fireside, a Division of Simon &
Schuster, Inc., ISBN 978-1-4165-4941-3

ISBN 978-1-84850-061-7

Printed in the UK by TJ International, Padstow, Cornwall.

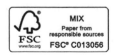

To all those out of rhythm who
are trying to find their beat

And to my patients,
whose journeys have guided my path

CONTENTS

PART I

Are You Spent?

Spent:

An Epidemic of Exhaustion

When the alarm rings, Emily groans and hits the snooze button. Lying there dreading the second ring, she feels dead on her feet before she is even on them. As she eases out of bed, she is aware of her stiff back, sore hips, and tight neck and shoulders. She shuffles to the bathroom to brush her teeth and, looking in the mirror, notices that her puffy eyes don't look as clear as they once did. Her hair and skin have become dull. She wonders if another cream or exercise regime might bring some life back into her. Then she heads to the kitchen for a bagel, a doughnut, maybe cereal with fruit and milk, or sometimes just a boost of caffeine. As she sips her coffee, she is assaulted with the daily TV or newspaper report of the latest tragedy, celebrity adventure, and clothes, cars, and products she should buy. Bolstered with caffeine, carbs, and sugar, or sometimes on an empty stomach, the daily scramble begins—whether it begins with going to work or getting the kids off to school, there are a multitude of responsibilities facing her. She heads out the door already haunted by guilt over things that will be left undone. But she soldiers on, diving into a day that is sure to be spent at a frantic pace—fending off and engaging with e-mails, phone calls, bills, employers and employees, children's schoolwork, family projects, and her husband's life.

Emily gets to work and her caffeine buzz might have her a little up, but an hour later she feels as if she has already been working for eight hours. Her thinking feels fuzzy. Her boss asks her a simple question, and even though somewhere in her brain she knows she has the answer, she can't think of it. These days her memory is unreliable. And so is her ability to concentrate—regular tasks take much longer to accomplish.

What does Emily do to deal with this debilitating combination of stress, fog, and fatigue? She does whatever it takes to get her through the day. She eats snacks full of sugar. She drinks—more coffee or soda. She smokes. She takes a tranquilizer. She exercises. She calls her therapist to up her antidepressant. But none of these "fixes" seems to last very long—a few hours or maybe a day. Maybe every once in a while she gets lucky and hits a combination that works for a week or so, but before she knows it, fatigue and stress are once again pounding on her front door.

At the end of the day, Emily drags herself home, too tired to take pleasure in her family, too beat to go out and enjoy the company of friends. In fact, just about everything feels like a chore these days. When the phone rings, it seems more like an imposition rather than an opportunity to connect. And nothing—from a bath to a day off work—seems to restore her. Things that used to energize her seem arduous or just supply a quick rush of adrenaline with no lasting sense of rejuvenation. And activities she used to enjoy—even sex—feel like too much effort. So Emily spends many of her evenings draped on her couch barely awake in front of the TV. Then, like a cruel joke, when it is time for bed, she can't fall asleep—no matter how exhausted she is. Or, if and when Emily finally does fall asleep, she doesn't sleep soundly. The cycle continues. Instead of refreshed and alert, she wakes up the following morning feeling groggy and tired.

After a few months of this seemingly endless fatigue, unexplainable physical aches, and a few colds in quick succession, Emily decides to see her doctor. After running some blood and other diagnostic tests, he tells her there is nothing wrong. He says that she is just getting older and hands her a prescription for the latest anti-inflammatory pill. So she goes to another physician, who tells her that she has a "chemical imbalance" and perhaps a new kind of sleeping pill or a different antidepressant drug might help. When she tells him she has tried all these pills in the last few months and is actually feeling worse, he says she needs a vacation. But she knows something is not right even though both doctors give her a clean bill of health, and that's when she comes to see me. I tell Emily that I know what this bone-weary, awful funk is because I see it all the time—and have been treating patients for it for more than twenty years.

Since I began practicing medicine in New York in the 1980s, I have noticed this alarming health trend. Despite being apparently disease-free and in the prime of their lives, people in their thirties, forties, and fifties have come to see me in disturbingly increasing numbers for help with similar complaints. An unbelievable 75 percent of the people I treat are overwhelmed, exhausted, and afflicted with this disorder that makes them feel decades older than their years. I call it Spent, because that is how you feel. You don't have enough wherewithal to live your life. You are running on empty. Your energy account is tapped out.

If you can identify with Emily's troubling picture and are wondering if you too are suffering from Spent, take this brief quiz.

ARE YOU SPENT?

1. Do you wake up in the morning and not feel refreshed?
2. Do you feel unusually tired most of the time?
3. Do you need coffee, soda, or sugary snacks to get going and keep going?
4. Although you feel physically exhausted, does your mind continue to race?
5. Do you feel as if you are aging too quickly?
6. Do you have gas, bloating, constipation, and/or indigestion?
7. Is it a struggle to lose weight in spite of dieting and exercise?
8. Do you have achy muscles and/or joints or tension in your body—particularly your neck and shoulders?
9. Do you have a diminished sex drive?
10. Do you often feel depressed or have trouble concentrating and focusing and remembering things?
11. Have you found that little or nothing seems to rejuvenate you?
12. Do you lack motivation to accomplish even small tasks?
13. Do you find that you get sick more frequently and that it takes longer to recover?

If you answered yes to more than three of these questions, you are more than likely Spent. As the name suggests, you are burned out—physically, mentally, and spiritually—and you need help. If you don't address this problem, you will continue to suffer and probably begin to feel even worse. The good news: this book is here to gently and safely guide you to a healthier, more vibrant, and happier you.

There Is a Solution

Over the last two decades, I have developed a program that has revived many thousands of people who seemed hopeless. I've witnessed countless people who've been transformed from weak, overwhelmed, sick, and tired to energized, inspired, strong, and profoundly healthy. My patients repeatedly tell me that after they've followed this program, their friends and colleagues suddenly start asking them what exactly have they done that has made them look so good—did they have a face-lift? Why are their eyes sparkling? Have they just returned from a great vacation? How did they lose weight?

Let me tell you right now, what you are feeling is *not* part of the "normal" aging process. Although you feel run-down and exhausted, it is within your power not only to make yourself feel better but quite possibly to feel better than you've ever felt. Moreover, this process of healing Spent is not as complicated and unpleasant as you might think. On the contrary, it is highly likely that once you incorporate this program into your life, you'll find so much to enjoy that you will become inspired and excited by your life. You might even end up inspiring others.

Getting Back into Rhythm

Each of us comes into the world endowed with essential energy. This energy operates as a kind of bank account and supplies us with the power to grow and regenerate ourselves daily. We are meant to supplement this original endowment of energy with what we can manufacture from eating, breathing, sleeping, learning, working, playing, and relationships. Each day we make withdrawals and deposits. But when the balance of the scales tips to our using more than we put back, we're in the red, with the prospect of getting further and further behind. Then we are forced to dip into our savings. When we continuously withdraw from our savings account, alarms begin to sound telling us that our survival is being challenged. These alarms are known to us as symptoms such as fatigue, apathy, depression, insomnia, brain fog, lowered resistance, stiffness, digestive problems, and signs of aging. These are our body's way of telling us that we are mentally, emotionally, and physically Spent. When we are Spent, our body is doing everything it can to tell us that it is time to slow down, rest, detoxify, repair, replenish, and restore.

Our bodies were not built to be sedentary or run marathons, exist on nearly no sleep, live without sun and nature, eat bizarre combinations of processed foods, or subsist on no-fat or no-carb diets. Nor were our brains wired to handle profound amounts of mental and emotional stress. We get Spent because our modern lifestyle has removed us from nature and we have become divorced from its rhythms and cycles.

We evolved over thousands of generations as beings who lived and worked in harmony with the seasons, and as a result these rhythms became imprinted in our genes. They are part of every aspect of our body's inner workings. Dr. Sidney Baker, one of the fathers of functional medicine, describes more than one hundred rhythms that form our internal body clock. This clock has what are called circadian rhythms, which reflect nature's twenty-four-hour cycle of day and night and govern most of our physiological processes.[1] "Circadian" comes from the Latin *circa,* meaning "about," and *diem,* or "day," thus "about a day." Each rhythm influences a unique aspect of body function, including body temperature, hormone levels, heart rate, blood pressure, even pain threshold. Every system in the body is affected by circadian rhythms.[2] And just as "official" clocks are set precisely to Greenwich Mean Time, our body clocks are set precisely to these natural rhythms. Science has shown clear patterns of brain wave activity, hormone production, enzyme production, cell regeneration, and other biological activities, each linked to these daily rhythms.[3]

As *Homo sapiens,* we are physically and mentally designed to eat natural and seasonal foods from our nearby environs and exercise in spurts— exert, rest, recover, exert, and so on. We are meant to have fresh air, sun, and water. We are built to sleep when the sun goes down and wake when it rises. And very few of us are living this way. Though I am not suggesting that everyone give up their homes and go live in a hut fashioned of sticks and mud, I firmly believe that if we don't move back in the direction of our genes, we will all ultimately end up Spent. In other words, we need to move back to our body's innate natural biochemical rhythms and genetic design because in our genes and biology we are still our ancient ancestors—yet we are living at a pace and rhythm that are completely foreign to our genes and biology. Fortunately, when prompted correctly with natural light and good food at the correct time, the right supplements, appropriate exercise, and exposure to nature, our genetic clocks can reset themselves.

How I Discovered the Importance of Rhythm

Soon after I graduated from medical school in Johannesburg, South Africa, where I grew up, I began treating patients in the rural areas of KwaNdebele. Although it was only about two hours north of Johannesburg, the biggest city in South Africa, it was like being in the middle of nowhere. Despite facing the harsh realities of poverty-stricken lives, the people didn't present symptoms of insomnia, depression, or anxiety. Women would carry their babies on their backs all day, walking long distances with buckets of water or other heavy loads balanced on their heads, yet they rarely came to the doctor complaining of back pain or fatigue. In many ways, this community was healthier than the patients I was seeing at my other job in a private practice in one of the wealthy suburbs of Johannesburg. Sure, they had some disease (mostly from poor sanitation and untreated water) and came to the hospital with broken bones or pneumonia, but they did not suffer from fatigue, headaches, digestive problems, or the general aches and pains that my more sophisticated urban patients did. Since there was no electricity, people were forced to live with the rhythms of nature. Day and night dictated what was done when, and being synchronous with the seasons was essential for survival. Community, music, and dance also played an integral role in bringing rhythm into their lives. It was during my time with these people that I began to be aware of the importance of nature's rhythm and its powerful impact on our health.

I wanted to bring what I had learned about these healthy communities living in touch with nature and one another in KwaNdebele to my patients in Johannesburg, who were a lot like Emily. As a young clinician who had recently finished medical school, my training focused upon hospital-based patients who were acutely sick or critically ill—heart attacks, acute asthma attacks, cancers, broken bones. These are the problems that Western medicine is designed to treat. But the subtle symptoms such as fatigue, anxiety, insomnia, and low-grade chronic complaints that I was seeing in my urban outpatients were not well addressed by my medical training. I found it very ironic that these vague complaints commonly expressed by urban patients were the very ones that conventional Western medicine does not have any good solutions for.

As I did not want to work in a hospital setting, I thought to myself, "There has to be a better way." I was trained to help people. I took the Hippocratic Oath, which declares, "First, do no harm." I felt that dispensing drugs was a quick fix, a Band-Aid solution that was not helping my patients in the long term and was potentially harmful. So I began what has become a lifelong journey to explore alternative methods to deeply, truly help people.

Soon after working in KwaNdebele, I emigrated to the United States. After doing the required internal medicine residency, I began a rigorous study of Chinese medicine, which turned my world inside out. Instead of symptoms being seen as something to suppress with drugs, they became a clue to some imbalance in the body—a sign that the body was out of rhythm. Within this picture, the role of the doctor was to re-create balance and restore rhythm, which, after my experience in rural South Africa, resonated with me. This completely different philosophical outlook led me to a radically new way of regarding and treating the body.

I learned that with acupuncture, it is possible to unblock congestion and restore flow, reestablishing a healthy homeostasis or balance in the body. Initially, this was a hard concept for me to grasp. But as I worked with more patients, I saw the difference between people who were in rhythm and balanced and those who were not. People who were in rhythm had a stronger pulse; clear eyes; a clean, healthy tongue; clear, robust skin; and were focused yet relaxed—they felt good, both to me and to themselves.

My Chinese medicine teachers taught me to see the body as a garden and myself, the doctor, as a gardener. When a plant is sick or not doing well, it is crucial to look at the environment in which the plant is growing: What is the quality of the soil? Is it getting enough nutrients? Does it have enough sun, water, and so on? Which is exactly how we are going to look at you in this book. As a creature of nature, you too need light, nutrients, and healthy soil to thrive.

On my journey, I also discovered functional medicine, where I learned about the importance of the environment and its effect on gene activity. I had been taught in medical school to think that your genes are carved in stone and that the diseases you get are determined by them. We now know that for the most part this is not true. The new science of epigenetics has shown that genetic activity is determined by your responses to the environment. In other words, how you live your life determines how your genes are expressed. You may have a genetic predisposition to a disease, but the environment you bathe your cells and genes in determines how those genes are expressed. This means that there are lots of potential versions of you. Whether you become Spent is determined by the unique way your genes interact with the many variables in their environment. So what you eat, how much chemical and toxic exposure you have had, what stresses you have tolerated, how you think, how much love you get, and how you move are *critical*. Like a computer, our cells, and therefore our organs, are programmable—their health is determined by what information they download from the outside and what information you feed them.

In both Chinese medicine and functional medicine, I also learned that one could improve the functioning of organs. This concept was never addressed in Western medicine; you had either a healthy liver or liver disease—nothing in between. Western medicine offered no ways to improve the function of the organs before they became diseased. In Chinese and functional medicine, one could use acupuncture, herbs, nutrition, supplements, certain breathing techniques, or exercise to improve the functioning of various organs as a means of treating and preventing disease. This meant that my treatments would not only provide immediate relief but also offer a lasting change for my patients. (To learn more about Chinese medicine or functional medicine, go to www.spentmd.com.)

But first I had to find the best means of merging all of these modalities—my Western training, my Chinese medicine and functional medicine studies—to foster enduring balance and rhythm. I became the ultimate guinea pig. Restorative yoga, interval training, alternative diets, juice fasts, supplements, tonics, meditations, dance, different types of body-work, healing with music, and sweats were all part of my experimenting. You name it, and I've probably tried it. Out of this personal research as well as from the many thousands of people who have been helped through my work, I developed a comprehensive system for getting people back into rhythm—and a more refined system for healing Spent.

Your Total Load

One of the most influential ideas I have come across in my research and that has shaped the way I practice and work with Spent is the concept of a person's *total load*. A person's total load is the total amount of physical, psychological, and environmental stress on his or her body. In the last thirty years, this total load on the human body has quadrupled. As I mentioned in my earlier discussion, our bodies were not genetically designed for this modern life load, making it much more difficult for us to stay healthy and avoid being Spent. On a daily basis, most of us don't get enough vital nutrients, sleep, or appropriate exercise. We sit too much, watch too much TV, and eat too much. And then there is the cocktail of hundreds of man-made toxins—from our cleaning products to the products we put on our skin to the chemicals in our food and water. Our natural habits have shifted from living close to and in sync with the earth to coming in contact with and consuming quantities of warping ingredients, confounding our ability to cope successfully. In an endless variety of ways, we are distorting our natural genetic blueprint for living.

The buildup of these multiple assaults on our bodies adds to our total load until a tipping point is reached and we become Spent. Everyone's tipping point is different, and now you have an opportunity to tip the balance in the other direction.

Some factors that add to our total load are within our control (diet, lifestyle choices), while some are ubiquitous and out of our sphere of influence (plastics in our environment, the air we breathe, the stimuli we encounter daily). This book is about taking charge of what we can change and those changes acting powerfully to rehabilitate us. It's about maximizing our adaptive capacities and turning ourselves around. You can literally lighten your load.

Actually, the fact that we are not all Spent is really a testament to how extraordinary our bodies are—their capacity to adapt and evolve. My philosophy is, if our bodies can adapt to this kind of toxic environment and survive, what would happen if we gave our bodies a garden to flourish in? Because there are so many factors that contribute to our total load and therefore our health and well-being, my program for healing Spent takes the gardener's approach: create—from the soil up—an environment in and around the body that will foster abundant health and growth. I look at the earth, the roots, trunk, limbs, encroaching weeds, lack of nutrients, potential poisons, water, light, air. And I make sure that everything going into and around the body is working to support your life and health. In this book, I will not only help you nourish yourself with the right food at the right time but also assess your physical activities and environment. I'll help you find ways to cope with the enormous mental and psychological stress that affects most modern lives. Even if we are doing everything right physically and dietwise, mental stress alone can bring on Spent. To calculate your total load, go to www.spentmd.com.

My program for healing Spent is a day-by-day guide to helping you regain your mind and body's natural rhythm. You will learn to work with your body's natural rhythms and not fight them. No matter how long your rhythms have been unbalanced, this is "a situation subject to change," as one of my patients says. No matter how sick you are, resetting and restoring rhythm is a completely doable—and enjoyable—process.

How We Will Work

Everyone's life is different. Everyone's body is different. And everyone heals differently. This is even more true when a person is Spent. A Spent body—no matter what kind of body it is—cannot endure quick, drastic changes, as this only throws the body even more out of rhythm. Rather than giving you an aggressive program of dos, don'ts, and shoulds, I am offering you a sane guide for how to heal over time. These suggestions are based on my almost thirty years of experience with Spent and patients like you, along with my constant engagement with the latest research and my relationships and conversations with some of the best practitioners around the world. The Spent program will help nudge you and your unique body back into rhythm.

Lao-tzu, the father of Taoism, said, "To attain knowledge, add things every day. To attain wisdom, remove things every day." This sums up my philosophy of medicine and is also a good way to look at and talk about treating Spent: removing and adding and adding and removing to help the body shift and find its natural balance and innate wisdom.

I've divided this book into forty-two digestible daily actions—Daily Beats—that will remove burdens from your body's total load and add things that will help your body heal more quickly and, most important, make you feel better. Over the course of the next six weeks, these Daily Beats will make the process of restoring your body and mind to their normal rhythm relatively easy. Some days we will remove, and some days we will add.

You may be wondering what exactly you will be removing and adding. Because Spent is multifaceted, we will be working to restore your mind and body from many angles, including sleep, diet, exercise, supplements, meditation, and relaxation. For instance, one exercise suggestion will be for you not to work out like a maniac. One relaxation suggestion is to listen to certain types of music, such as reggae or certain classical compositions. This kind of music physiologically entrains your body to slow down and relax. Dietwise, I will give you an in-depth preview of the eating program in the next chapter. But for now, know that I will be suggesting that you eat more whole, organic foods and cut out white sugar. This said, there will be absolutely no calorie or fat counting.

At the end of each of these Daily Beats, there is a Pulse section. This section is your backup, helping you integrate each suggestion into your life. Each suggestion will be repeated for a few days to help you find your pace. And then I will follow up a few times in the following days and weeks so that you can make this part of the program and healing your own. For instance, when I ask you to make a dietary change in the program, I will include that new change in the Pulse for several days in a row, to help get you started, and then I will give you a few days to play with it before I come back and talk about it again. New Beats are in bold type and indicated by ●. Repeat Beats are indicated by ○. After the Pulse, there is a Sleep Beat section, which is focused on your sleep life. How you sleep is as important as how you live during your waking hours. When we are Spent, one of our essential needs is sound sleep. These sleep recommendations will teach you how to improve your bedtime habits so that you will truly sleep like a baby. As with the Pulse, the Sleep Beat will remind you of new sleep tips for a few days and then give you a few days to explore and play with the suggestions before I ask you to think about them again.

Though I have organized these suggestions and sections for adding and subtracting into a six-week schedule, go at your own pace. If the program feels great, follow each beat by the calendar day. If you find you are getting overwhelmed, rather than giving up completely, stay on whatever day you're on, "shop around" a little in the book for something that looks as if it will feel *really* good, and stay there for a while. This said, I have been honing this system for years, and the add and remove days have been carefully calibrated so that you will not take too much out or add too much, thus taxing your body even more. This program is about relieving stress and restoring energy, not giving you more to do and making you even more exhausted. Listen to your life and body. For instance, if you get five actions done in a row and then have to go on a business trip or your child gets sick, do your best to adhere to the program, but don't be obsessive about it.

Adhering to the eating program will be beneficial and, more than likely, easier. For instance, I will be asking you to give up caffeine for three or four weeks, which can be excruciating unless you do so in the suggested phases and with the other suggested actions to support your body and mind. And once you're off the stuff, you'll feel so much better that you will probably stay off it.

Healing Spent is as much about listening and paying attention to the ebb and flow of your life as it is about a specific diet or exercise. At first you might not even know what I mean by "listening to your body," but if you take the suggestions one day at a time, you will most likely find out that you can hear your own rhythm, the beat that your body and mind need to feel healthy and strong again.

Start where you are. Take an action. Listen. Pause if you need to. Come back to the work. Maybe begin again or start where you left off. The best results will come with effort, and that part is your responsibility. If you falter, don't use this as an opportunity to beat yourself up. Practice shrugging your shoulders and saying "oh well," and get back on the horse. In fact, if you learn only that, you'll be way ahead of the game. The results will come, you can be assured of that. Your body, mind, and spirit will heal. And you will soon be living in a healthy home again.

This process of returning to your natural genetic rhythm is not a thirty-day lose-weight, look-great-for-a-party trick. It is about making a profound change. A patient described how the process felt to her this way: it was as if her body were a glass of muddy water and every day we stirred it up, took out a teaspoon, and added a teaspoon of fresh pure water. Each day the glass became a little clearer, and eventually she had a glass of fresh, sparkling water.

In the words of Khalil Gibran, "You work that you may keep pace with the earth and the soul of the earth. For to be idle is to become a stranger unto the seasons, and to step out of life's procession." So let's get to work to get back into life's procession. And let's see what happens when you give your body a garden to flourish in and get its natural rhythm back. I think you will be astounded by how good you will feel before you are even halfway through.

Prepare

As I mentioned in the introduction, one of the key aspects of restoring your body to its natural rhythm is proper nourishment. This chapter is devoted to helping you prepare your kitchen for the Spent program—specifically for my restorative eating program. Avoiding the foods I suggest will give your digestive system a much-needed rest, which will not only help your body's ability to process food and absorb it more efficiently but also help nearly every other system, organ, and bodily function get back into rhythm.

Eat to Beat Feeling Spent: Restorative Eating

When I review the habits, lifestyle, and symptoms of any of my patients who are Spent, I almost always see a pattern of profound nutritional depletion. I have therefore designed a program that will build a resource of energy the likes of which you probably haven't experienced in years. The bad news: you will have to give up comforts like caffeine, sugar, bread, and processed foods for a while. But this is not—I repeat, *not*—about deprivation. In fact, it is quite the opposite. Restorative eating and healing Spent is about abundance. As I've said, there is no calorie counting or portion control. Restorative eating is about feeding yourself delicious, high-quality foods and ultimately supporting and replenishing your overwhelmed systems. There are powerful foods and treats that will replace what's been hurting you with what can heal you.

Anyone who's ever dieted to lose weight knows that the focus has swung in the last few years from low-fat to low-carb. Neither of these approaches will help you recover from Spent (for that matter, I question how useful these approaches are for long-term weight loss, too). Instead, I want you to focus on the *quality* of the fats and carbs you eat and make sure that every bite contains plenty of healthy nutrients and as few added chemicals or toxins as possible. In fact—and this may shock you—I'm convinced that it's much more important to pay attention to the *quality* of fats, carbs, and protein than to the *quantity* of these foods.

For most of my patients, the Spent restorative eating program is the heart of the healing process. Over the course of six weeks, I essentially revolutionize what they eat, when they eat, and how they eat. Because if the what, when, and how are not all in sync with one another, the body's eating rhythm is off and they are not able to absorb and process food properly. And, as you know, when our body is not getting appropriate nourishment, we get sick.

Likewise, over the course of the next six weeks, I will be asking you to rethink what, when, and how you eat. Consequently, there will be days when I ask you to begin taking a food out of your diet for the duration of the six weeks. Note that what food I remove and when I take it out depend entirely on how harmful and Spent-causing the food is. For instance, I will ask you to take processed sugars out immediately and for the entire six weeks, whereas I will ask you to limit your soy consumption for only a few weeks. I consider refined sugars to be incredibly toxic and Spent-inducing and soy just mildly problematic.

As I mentioned in my introduction, the Spent restorative eating program doesn't just take foods out. There will be days when I will ask you to add certain foods or supplements to your diet, as I consider these to be incredibly powerful tools for healing the digestive system and Spent. For example, one of the reasons I suggest that people who are Spent drink smoothies is that there is less for the digestive system to break down. Less work for the body. More energy for you.

And there will be days when I will ask you to look at how and when you are eating—Standing alone in your kitchen at ten at night? Wolfing down food with friends, trying to make a movie? As you can imagine, neither of these practices is great for a Spent body.

As with all of my recommendations, your success will depend on making this eating plan work for you—and for your family, if that's possible and appropriate. The plan is simple, flexible, and natural. I don't think you'll be shocked to see organic whole foods and a bare minimum of prepared or processed foods on the eating plan, which can accommodate both vegetarians and carnivores. But because preparing whole foods can take a little more time, and because most of you are very busy people (although I'm trying to slow you down), part of this program is dedicated to creating a system that makes it easy to grab the foods you love when you need them. The plan also teaches you how to know what types of food you need at different times of the day (you need different nutrients in the morning, noon, and night) and at different times of your life (such as when you are early in this recovery or severely stressed versus when you are in the maintenance phase). Strict adherence to a planned diet isn't your goal—your goal is to give yourself the nutritional resources you need to feel better than you've ever felt before.

Cooking and preparing meals for Spent is not just about specific foods or recipes; it is a strategy to make delicious, simple, and healthy food by being properly prepared and organized. A well-stocked pantry and fridge are key, as is planning your meals in advance so that no matter how Spent you feel, you will still be able to put together three tasty, healthy meals each day. The following sections are a guide to help you prepare your kitchen for the restorative eating portion of the book. It is important to prepare ahead, as I will most likely be taking some of the staples of your diet out of your kitchen and I want you always to have something around that you can eat and enjoy.

First Things First: Digestion

Before we go to your kitchen, we need to talk about your body. I can't talk about food, eating, and nourishing the body without first talking about digestion. While many of my Spent patients don't come in complaining of digestive symptoms, more often than not, faulty digestion is one of their most significant problems. The majority of them don't realize that their digestive systems have slowly eroded and aren't functioning optimally.

Many of us have become used to mild indigestion, irritated bowels, bloating, and/or gas and think they are a normal part of aging. We see them as an inevitable nuisance rather than a real issue that needs to be addressed. Walk down the aisles of any drugstore or supermarket, and you will see hundreds of over-the-counter digestion "remedies" for gas, diarrhea, and indigestion. In fact in 2005, two of the four top-selling drugs in the United States were for digestive problems.[1] Unfortunately, these drugs, as with most drugs, treat only the symptoms and don't heal the real problem.

What you really want is a fully functioning digestive system so that you digest and absorb your food's vital nutrients. Because no matter how healthily you eat, if your digestive system does not work well, your food does not nourish you well. You want your food to actually feed you.

One common problem with a Spent digestive system is that the lining of the gut (your digestive system) is damaged. The gut's lining is extremely thin, often just one cell thick. This damage can be extremely problematic because 70 to 80 percent of your immune system is found in your digestive tract. When this delicate lining is damaged or worn down by a poor diet or large food particles, bacteria and toxins that should normally stay in your gut's inner tube pass through it into the bloodstream, where the immune system must deal with them. These leaking particles tax your immune system. Thus, with a poorly functioning digestive system, you don't just get digestive symptoms, you also get an exhausted immune system. To add insult to injury, you can also get pain. An overactive immune system can lead to inflammation in the body. Just think of the swelling that occurs around a cut on your hand. Your immune system creates the same kind of swelling to fight hurt and unhealthy cells inside your body. This is one of the reasons why your body feels so cranky and achy when you are Spent.

Another reason for keeping your digestion in good shape is the ecosystem of bacterial flora, the trillions of bugs that reside in your gut. There are more than five hundred species of bacteria in your gut, most of them "good guys," helping you digest your food, produce vitamins, excrete toxins, regulate hormones, and generally keep your gut healthy and balanced. These functions are impaired when there are too many of the "bad guys" and not enough of the "good guys." But most important, an imbalance in the flora can damage the delicate gut lining and lead to Spent. Antibiotics are just one environmental element that can destroy the balance between good and bad. These "bad guys" can also move into areas where they shouldn't be (such as the small intestine, which normally does not contain bacteria) and cause digestive problems that can also lead to Spent.

A relatively unknown fact is that your gut actually functions like a second brain. More than half of your body's nerve cells are located in your gut. Dr. Michael Gershon, a professor at New York City's Columbia-Presbyterian Medical Center and author of *The Second Brain,* refers to the entire gastrointestinal system as "the body's second nervous system." According to Dr. Gershon, the brain is not the only place in the body that has lots of neurotransmitters. There are a hundred million neurotransmitters lining the length of the gut, which is about the same number found in the brain.[2] Nearly every brain-regulating chemical found in your brain is also found in your gut's brain—including both hormones and neurotransmitters. In fact, the vast majority of serotonin, one of the better-known neurotransmitters in the body, is made in the gut, not the brain. Dr. Gershon points out that our brain and gut mirror each other so much that both have natural ninety-minute "sleep cycles." In the brain, slow-wave sleep is interrupted by periods of rapid eye movement (REM) sleep, during which dreams occur. The gut has corresponding ninety-minute cycles of slow-wave muscle contractions. As with the brain's REM sleep intervals, these cycles are interrupted by corresponding short bursts of rapid muscle movement. Like everything else in the body, there is a rhythm to digestion.

Of course, the two brains are connected and affect each other. Mental stress can upset your digestion, and digestive stress can cause anxiety and depression and affect your moods in general. How we eat has a physiological effect on how we feel.

Beyond the health of the gut, a relatively new field of study called nutrigenomics offers what I consider an even more potent argument for eating wholesome foods. Nutrigenomics examines the interactions among foods and specific genes that regulate the risk of common chronic diseases, including type 2 diabetes, obesity, heart disease, stroke, and certain cancers. Nutrigenomics' core premise is that the influence of diet on health is related to your unique genetic makeup. Nutrigenomics tells us that food contains "hidden instructions," which are communicated directly to your genes. Armed with this information, your genes influence various metabolic actions and millions of critical biological processes, including cholesterol levels, aging, hormone regulation, weight gain and loss, and much more.

Once you understand that food is "data" that the body uses to direct the complex actions that keep us vibrantly alive, it's easy to understand that loading up on junk food is like taking the fast lane to a giant system failure—meaning Spent and its tiresome symptoms.

When you think about it, it makes perfect sense. As I said in the introduction, our genes evolved to accept and depend upon whole foods for our survival over countless generations. Since our genes are very similar to those of our Paleolithic ancestors, they are not well adapted to cereal grains, sugar, factory farmed meats, and pasteurized dairy foods. In particular, our genes aren't adapted to processed foods and their weird chemical molecules, unhealthy fats, refined carbohydrates, and potentially toxic chemicals. Your immune system treats these unnatural molecules the same way it treats invaders such as pollens, bacteria, and viruses, though in a subtler way: it slowly mounts a response against them that triggers inflammation and other reactions aimed at removing or containing the invaders.

The other function of the body that is particularly taxed by these unhealthy foods is that of your hormones. We'll talk about hormones in greater depth later. But for now, you need to know that your hormones are the chemicals that govern your body, from your metabolism to your moods and sex drive. These hormonal systems are very sensitive and already have enough to do to keep your body up and running. So when you overwhelm your body with sugars or chemicals, your body's hormonal systems not only have to accomplish their daily tasks but now have an extra job to do: restore balance in the body after it has been attacked by a toxic substance. Over time, these reactions to foreign chemicals can create disease processes such as heart disease, cancer, arthritis, gastrointestinal problems, and Spent.

Now that we have a sense of some of the factors that commonly cause damage to our gut, genes, and hormones and that can lead to feeling Spent, we can begin to heal.

Welcome to Our Kitchen

Like you, my wife, Janice, and I have busy lives. But for the last twenty years we have become more and more committed to eating fresh, organic, nourishing food on a daily basis. In this time, we have spent many hours together talking about how we eat and how to improve our approach to cooking and eating. Nowadays, we have a refined system for shopping, chopping, and cooking, along with our favorite recipes and key pantry items that I will share with you in the course of the program. Nothing we are asking you to do is just a concept. These are road-tested, tongue-tested, time-tested ways of approaching shopping, cooking, and eating that are truly simple, flexible, and natural.

THE LIPMANS' FIVE RULES
FOR COOKING AND EATING

1. Get organized. Check your pantry to see what ingredients you have and don't have, using the lists beginning on page 30 as your guide.

2. Think ahead. Look at the recipes, decide what you will make over the course of the next week, and prepare a shopping list. It is also a good idea to sometimes choose recipes that you can double so that you can "cook once and use twice," that is, the leftovers can be incorporated into a meal for the next day.

3. Prepare ahead. The more preparation you can do in advance, the less work there will be to do later. At our house, this means getting home from the market and dedicating some time to preparing our food. We make salad dressings, marinades, a grain salad, or soup and spend an hour or so cutting up, dicing, or shredding ingredients that can be kept in airtight containers for a couple of days and stored in the fridge, ready to use when we need them. For example, we cut up carrots, celery, cauliflower, broccoli, peppers, and cabbage and store them in airtight glass containers. We

do not wash them until we are ready to use them. Prepackaged and prewashed salad greens are also a great time saver. Many fresh vegetables can also be prepared in advance by steaming, blanching, or roasting. We then use these vegetables in salads or stir-fries or reheat them later. Vegetables such as cauliflower, butternut squash, asparagus, peppers, and broccoli are also available precut in many markets, and these can be roasted at the same time that you prepare the rest of your meal. Or they can be used in a stir-fry or salad. (If you use any prepackaged produce, please remember to check the "use by" date to ensure freshness.)

4. Be creative. Many of the recipes can be adapted according to your own personal tastes and preferences and the availability of ingredients. Each season presents an opportunity to make changes in what we eat. Take advantage of what's seasonal and abundant in your area.

5. Enjoy your food. Don't stand by the kitchen sink or sit hunched on the edge of your couch with the TV blaring as you scarf down food. Set a place for yourself at a table. Sit down. Relax. Take small bites. Chew your food. Take pleasure in eating. Savor the taste. Appreciate the fact that you are fueling your mind and body. Share your meal with loved ones or friends.

THE FOUR FOOD GROUPS

The focus of the restorative eating plan is to increase the consumption of foods that nourish our bodies and to limit or stop eating the foods that hurt our bodies—mentally, digestively, and genetically. To help you distinguish among the good, the bad, and the ugly, I have divided foods into four groups:

1. Eat as much as you like. Eat as much of these foods as you like, as frequently as possible. These are my Spent Superfoods. You should eat several servings or more every day because they're especially dense in phytochemicals and other nutrients that help

battle Spent. Phytochemicals are the substances that give your fruits and vegetables their taste, smell, and color. These chemicals also work to protect the plant and anything that consumes it (for example, you) from harmful diseases and bacteria.

2. Eat in moderation. If possible, limit these foods to one serving or at most two servings a day while on the program. When you feel better, you can eat them more frequently. I'm not saying that these foods are unhealthy, but because many of them eventually turn into sugar in your body, you need to cut back on them as you begin your recovery. Although I recommend grass-fed meats and organic poultry, I appreciate that they are more expensive and not always available. As an alternative, please choose skinless poultry and the leanest cuts of meat available. The same holds true with the fish listed here. Although some of these fish can be quite contaminated with mercury, I include them to broaden the choices.

3. Avoid while on the program. Avoid these foods as much as possible during the program. As you recover and enter the maintenance phase, you may be able to eat a serving or two of these foods per week, depending on your individual constitution—some people can tolerate them, others can't. But I still do not recommend eating them regularly or in large amounts even when you're better; I believe these foods can, over time, contribute to Spent.

4. Avoid completely. These foods shouldn't be on anyone's regular diet, and if you're Spent, you should ban them as completely as you can. Though an occasional small indulgence won't hurt, especially after you're feeling better, the accumulation of these unhealthy foods in your system contributes to Spent and will slow or prevent your recovery.

The point of these four food groups is to help you learn to make the distinction between pure food (is grown, goes bad if not refrigerated or has a limited shelf life, is vibrantly colored, has its own natural flavor, is con-

nected to the land, has little or no packaging or labels a\
low profit margins) and food substances (are manufactured\
are packaged, contain artificial flavors, and have no connectic\
and a much larger profit margin). Pure foods include fruit\
whole grains, grass-fed meats, poultry, and wild-caught fish\
stances include any food products that have been created and pr ___ssed by
factories—breads, snack foods, salad dressings, frozen meals, and so on. *The
more pure food you eat, the better you will feel.*

We have put together an extensive list of each of these food groups
along with a wonderful collection of recipes in the Recipes for Renewal
section in the back of this book. As you might guess, these recipes feature
and promote pure food eating and cooking. You can find Recipes for Renewal beginning on page 268. (For a more extensive collection of healing
recipes, go to www.spentmd.com.) Peruse these and use them at your
pleasure. But for now, let's just get your pantry and kitchen ready for the
first week of the Spent program.

Clean Out, Stock Up, and Supply

In many ways, preparing for restorative eating is like packing for a trip,
which I personally hate. I never take the right number of socks and always
wonder if the hotel will supply soap or if I should pack some. This is why I
have given you the most thorough packing list I could possibly think of. As
you will see and experience, it is a bit over the top, but I decided I'd rather
err on the side of caution, particularly for my fellow packing haters. If
these next few pages seem like ridiculous hand-holding or total common
sense to you, blaze through and don't listen to my rants and raves about
chemicals and the benefits of spices. But if you are more like me and like
to have a list, embrace it. Everything is here for you. I have left nothing
out, so that, at least for this trip, you will have a perfectly packed suitcase.

To prepare for the program, there are three things you must do: *clean
out, stock up, and supply.* Please know that I realize these three steps may take
a few days. My suggestion is to carve out a weekend day to clean and shop.
But again, do this at your own pace and when you are ready. If you are
really tired and sick, you might ask a friend, your partner, or even your

and are well known to contribute to poor cardiovascular health and heart disease, not to mention nervous system disorders.

Artificial sweeteners, such as aspartame (NutraSweet and Equal), saccharin (Sweet'N Low), sucralose (Splenda) and acesulfame K. None has undergone long-term epidemiological studies on humans, and their health record is dubious at best. The Food and Drug Administration (FDA) approved sucralose for human consumption after only two published trials on humans, which had a total of thirty-six subjects. Although it is marketed as "Made from sugar so it tastes like sugar," it is more chemically similar to DDT.[3] Aspartame alone has more than ninety-two possible side effects. For more information, see www.sweetpoison.com. By the way, this means you should toss out or donate all of your soda and diet soda, not simply because of the chemical sweeteners they contain but because they are highly acidic drinks that disrupt the acid/alkaline balance in the human body. This disruption, in turn, causes your body to lose bone mass as it leaches calcium from your bones to offset the acid in your diet.

High-fructose corn syrup (HFCS), which is especially dangerous. Americans actually consume more HFCS than sugar. Research has shown that high-fructose corn syrup goes directly to the liver, releasing enzymes that instruct the body to store fat. Believe it or not, this can be found in some seemingly healthy foods—many flavored yogurts, granola bars, energy bars, and breakfast cereals contain HFCS.

Look for all other **refined sugars** in all their forms on the ingredients label, as manufacturers try to trick you into thinking their foods do not contain a lot of sugar. The following are various versions of refined sugar: cane sugar, dried cane syrup, brown sugar, beet sugar, date sugar, grape sugar, glucose, sucrose, maltose, maltodextrin, dextran, dextrose, sorbitol, corn syrup, fructose, high-fructose corn syrup, corn sugar, fruit juice, fruit juice concentrate, barley malt, caramel, carob syrup, and sorghum syrup.

Look at your breakfast cereals, white breads, salad dressing, pasta sauces, yogurts, granola and health bars, canned fruits, and so on.

Sodium nitrite and sodium nitrate, found in most packaged meat products and deli meats. They are precursor chemicals to powerful carcinogenic compounds that are well known to contribute to cancers of the digestive system. If you have packaged or factory-farmed meat—hot dogs, lunch meats, any meat or poultry that is not labeled "organic"—and can't bear to throw it out, eat it. But then, the next time you are at the market, buy grass-fed meat and organic poultry.

Monosodium glutamate (MSG), found in many "instant meals," frozen dinners, packaged meats, canned soups, soup stocks, salad dressings, soy sauces, spice mixes, flavorings, and seasonings. It is a commonly used seasoning in many restaurants too. If you see the words "sodium caseinate," "hydrolyzed protein," "autolyzed yeast," or "yeast extract" on a product's label, you can assume that the product contains some amount of MSG. It is known to be an excitotoxin, which means it damages nerve cells. Animal studies have also shown that it causes damage to the brain.

Also ax anything that has the following **additives**—a study published in *The Lancet* in September 2007 found that common food additives and colorings can increase hyperactive behavior in children.[4] Remember: the more chemicals you put into your body, the more they add to your toxic load and the more it will slowly wear your system down and lead to Spent. According to the Center for Science in the Public Interest, these food additives are harmful in the following ways:[5]

Sulfites (sulfur dioxide and sodium bisulfite), found in dried fruits. They commonly cause allergies.

Potassium bromate, found in factory-made breads. It is banned from use in food products in Europe, Canada, and most other countries, including China.

Preservatives (such as BHA, BHT, TBHQ), found in some
butter, meats, cereals, chewing gum, baked goods, snack
foods, dehydrated potatoes, and beer. Some studies show they
cause cancer in animals.

Artificial colors (such as FD&C Red No. 3, Yellow Nos. 5 and 6,
Blue Nos. 1 and 2), found in soda, sports drinks, and gelatin
desserts. Most artificial colorings are synthetic chemicals that
do not occur in nature and are used almost solely in foods of
low nutritional value.

Artificial fats (such as olestra), found in snack foods. Olestra
reduces the body's ability to absorb fat-soluble carotenoids
(such as alpha- and beta-carotene, lycopene, lutein, and
canthaxanthin) from fruits and vegetables, which reduce the
risk of cancer and heart disease.

Any other processed food. Processed foods are anything not produced in nature: quick or instant grains, meals in a package, box,
or can, factory-produced breads, dinner mixes, frozen meals. And
look out for snack foods, even ones that claim they are healthy
and sugar-free.

After you have gone through this list, take a final sweep. It does not
belong in your pantry or future shopping basket if:

- *The ingredient list is long*
- *The print is too fine*
- *You don't recognize more than two or three names*
- *There are too many names you can't pronounce*
- *There are too many ingredients your grandmother wouldn't have used*

These suggestions may sound funny, but they are great rules of thumb.
**Remember, the longer the ingredients label, the further away
the food is from nature and therefore the less healthy it is.** Read
ingredients lists before buying foods, and if you discover chemical names
that you can't pronounce, throw the food out and don't buy it again! Tak-

ing these chemicals, additives, processed foods, and junk food out of your house and life will drastically decrease your body's burden of toxicity. The less your body sees of these foods, the better you will feel.

Stock Your Kitchen

Now that your cupboards are nearly bare, it is time to fill them up with pure foods that will help heal Spent.

As I have already mentioned, there are certain foods that I call Spent Superfoods. These are the foods that you should stock and eat several servings or more of every day because they will nourish you appropriately to help defeat Spent.

Here I am giving you an abbreviated version of the full list, which is on page 260. The main purpose of today's list and subsequent grocery store visit is to get your pantry in order and begin our ongoing conversation about what you are eating and how you are preparing your meals. For greater ease, I've also put this list on my Web site. Go to www.spentmd .com, where you can download it and take it with you shopping. Additionally, the Web site has a list of the supplements you might need for the program—particularly a whey protein powder, a greens powder, and glutamine, which I suggest using during the first week.

PANTRY BASICS

Let's begin at the beginning by building your spice cabinet. Nothing replaces the aroma and aliveness of fresh herbs and spices. However, in most instances, fresh can be substituted with a good-quality (preferably nonirradiated) dried version. Keeping a supply of these in your pantry will allow you to make most of the recipes in this book without needing some unusual ingredient.

Arrowroot	*Cayenne pepper*
Basil	*Ground red chili powder*
Bay leaves	*Ground cinnamon*

Ground coriander

Ground cumin

Curry powder

Garam masala

Garlic powder

Ground ginger

Mint

Mustard powder

Oregano

Paprika

Pepper (black and white)

Red pepper flakes

Rosemary

Sea salt (coarse and fine)

Ground thyme

Ground turmeric

Optional extras

Gomasio

Sea salt with sea vegetables

These optional extras are nice to sprinkle on steamed or sautéed vegetables.

PANTRY STAPLES

In addition to herbs and spices, some good-quality staples are an essential part of any well-stocked pantry.

Organic canned beans

Organic chicken stock

Organic dried lentils (red and brown)

Canned wild salmon

Sardines in olive oil

Organic canned tomatoes (whole, peeled, diced, crushed)

Organic canned tomato paste

Sundried tomatoes in olive oil

Organic vegetable stock

Olives

There are some wonderful organic brands—Eden Foods, Muir Glen, Westbrae Natural, Pacific Natural Foods, and Imagine Foods—and both Trader Joe's and Whole Foods Market have their own-label organic products as well.

GRAINS

Amaranth

Steel-cut oats (not fast-cooking or instant)

Quinoa

Brown rice (short-grain and long-grain)

Brown rice pasta   Wild rice

Again, buy organic when you can.

CONDIMENTS

Agave syrup   Whole-grain mustard
Mirin   Soy sauce (get wheat-free and
Dijon-style mustard   low-sodium)

OILS

Coconut oil   Sesame oil and toasted sesame oil
Extra-virgin olive oil   for occasional use in stir-fries
                                        (optional)

VINEGAR

Balsamic vinegar   White wine vinegar
Red wine vinegar

SMOOTHIE INGREDIENTS

I'll talk more about smoothies in your first week, but you will need these
ingredients almost immediately, so please make sure you have them.

Almond milk (unsweetened)   Organic flaxseed oil
Rice milk (unsweetened) (if you   Vanilla or plain whey protein
    can't get almond milk)   powder (see www.spentmd.
Organic frozen blueberries,   com for my favorite brands)
    strawberries, mixed   A super green powdered product
    berries, cherries, pineapples,   (see www.spentmd.com
    peaches, mangoes   for my favorite brands)
Coconut water (if available)   Raw and unsalted almond butter

Tahini (sesame paste) Vanilla extract

Unsweetened cocoa powder

VEGETABLES

Asparagus   Kale

Avocado (actually a fruit)   Mushrooms

Bok choy   Olives

Broccoli   Onions

Brussels sprouts   Spinach

Cabbage (green and red)   Swiss chard

Carrots   Tomatoes (actually a fruit)

Cauliflower   Watercress

Celery

FRUITS

Blackberries   Pomegranates

Blueberries   Raspberries

Coconut   Strawberries

Kiwifruit

DRIED FRUITS FOR TRAIL MIX (ORGANIC IF POSSIBLE)

Dried unsulfured apricots   Dried chopped and unsweetened

Dried unsweetened shredded   dates

  coconut

NUTS AND SEEDS

Nuts should be bought raw and unsalted. Nuts that are already roasted have been roasted at such high temperatures that the valuable oils are degraded. If you like roasted nuts, you can slow-roast them in your toaster oven at 160° to 175° F. for 15 to 20 minutes.

Raw almonds

Raw brazil nuts

Raw cashew nuts

Ground flaxseeds

Raw pecans

Raw pumpkin seeds

Raw sesame seeds

Raw sunflower seeds

Raw walnuts

FISH

Anchovies

Black cod (sablefish)

Wild salmon (fresh and canned)

Canned sardines in olive oil

ORGANIC EGGS, MEAT, AND POULTRY

Organic eggs

Organic or free-range chicken and turkey

Grass-fed meat

SPECIALTY FOODS

Dark chocolate—70% to 85%

Cocoa nibs

Shopping Guidelines

Before you head out to the market, book in hand or, even easier, with your downloaded list, I have a few thoughts about shopping for your groceries. Downloads are available at www.spentmd.com.

1. Make a list.
2. Don't go shopping when you are hungry. Have a good meal before you go shopping.
3. Do your shopping in the outer aisles—produce, meats, fish, eggs. The inner aisles are usually full of processed foods, the ones full of sugar, trans fats, and other preservatives so their shelf life will be longer.

4. Remember, as a general rule, if there are ingredients that you can't recognize, pronounce, or spell, you probably should not be putting them into your body.

5. Be wary of "all natural." Although I am recommending an all-natural way of eating, "all natural" on a label is meaningless, as these foods are often high in sugars.

6. If you do buy a food in a box, choose one with five ingredients or fewer, none you can't pronounce, and no cartoon characters.

7. Select fruits and vegetables in a wide variety of colors.

8. Buy organic fruits and vegetables whenever you can, preferably locally grown. If that is not possible, at least avoid those that are most likely to be contaminated with pesticides. The Web site www.foodnews.org features the twelve fruits and veggies with the most and least pesticides so you'll know which ones to buy organic and which conventionally grown ones are okay when organic isn't available.

9. Buy fresh foods whenever possible—the fresher the food, the more nutritious. Fresh foods are better than frozen foods, but frozen foods are better than canned foods.

10. When buying meats, look for grass-fed meats and free-range poultry. Organic meats and poultry without hormones and antibiotics would be next best; if you can't find them, for meats get lean cuts, and for poultry remove the skin because toxins are stored in the fat.

11. Limit fish with a high mercury content (see page 171), and remember that ocean-caught fish are generally better than farm-raised fish, which are usually laden with PCBs (polychlorinated biphenyls). PCBs have been linked to reproductive problems, cancer, and immune and endocrine system disorders, among other issues.

12. Most important, *read the label*. Although most of the foods you are going to be choosing and eating don't actually have labels because they are from nature—fruits, vegetables, grass-fed meats, fish, nuts, seeds, and legumes—obviously you are also going to have to eat some food with labels. So it is important to continue

to read them, religiously looking out for the poisonous ingredients we just threw out:

- *Partially hydrogenated or hydrogenated fats and oils*
- *Artificial sweeteners*
- *High-fructose corn syrup and other refined sugars*
- *Sodium nitrite and sodium nitrate*
- *Monosodium glutamate (MSG)*
- *Sulfites (sulfur dioxide and sodium bisulfite)*
- *Potassium bromate*
- *Preservatives (such as BHA, BHT, TBHQ)*
- *Artificial colors (such as FD&C Red No. 3, Yellow Nos. 5 and 6, Blue Nos. 1 and 2)*
- *Artificial fats (such as olestra)*

A few more thoughts about your first few shopping trips:

1. In addition to the general list, you may want to choose a few recipes from the back of the book or from a more extensive collection at www.spentmd.com that sound good to you and you think you might want to try in the next week. Make sure you add all the ingredients for these recipes to your shopping list. My favorite feature that Janice and I have developed is the idea of a home salad bar, where you think of your refrigerator as your very own salad bar. You stock it with separate containers of different ingredients—organic greens and chopped-up organic vegetables, grilled and diced organic chicken or meat, a delicious salad dressing. This way you can easily mix and match whatever you want and quickly put together a delicious, nutrient-dense meal. This is a huge time and energy saver.

2. Give yourself time at the market. Whether we know it or not, we are programmed to move through our particular stores in a particular way. While you are healing from Spent, I will ask you to find new foods and read the labels of foods you previously bought to ensure that they are not harmful. Therefore, initially food shopping may take a little more time and attention than it did in the past.

3. Remember that not all food at the market is really food. Supermarkets provide a wonderful service, but remember, they are there to make money. In her book *What to Eat,* Marion Nestle, a highly regarded nutrition professor, explains that supermarkets' profits are in the junk food. These fancy, colorful, "miracle" chemicalized products are enticing, tasty, convenient, and often addictive.[6] They distract us from what we should be eating—whole fresh foods from nature. We are influenced by attractive advertising, smart packaging, and the clever placement of these products in the stores. A clean, fresh whole-foods diet contains fewer antibiotics, hormones, pesticides, hydrogenated fats, additives, preservatives, chemical sweeteners, and other chemicals and therefore decreases the toxic load on your body. This will make you more vital and less Spent.

Once again, make sure the bulk of your foods don't have labels!

Supply Your Kitchen

The last thing you need to do to prepare for my restorative eating program is to make sure that you have most of the following kitchen tools—particularly a blender—so that you can make all the delicious recipes we provide. Having the right tools is essential to easy food preparation.

It's easy to be seduced by different kitchen gadgets that, once bought, are often left lying unused in the kitchen drawer. We try to keep our kitchen tools reasonably basic, with a few extras. Here are some of our favorites in no particular order:

A blender, essential for smoothies

A stick blender, aka immersion blender, which is great for pureeing directly in the pot

A food processor

A salad spinner

A set of measuring cups and spoons

Tongs

A timer

A chopping board (maybe one big one and one small one)

A good set of kitchen knives for chopping, peeling, slicing, and dicing	*A cast-iron grill pan*
	A whisk or egg beater
	A strainer
Kitchen scissors	*A pepper mill*
A hand grater	*A set of good cooking pots and sauté pans (for stir-fries, or a wok if you prefer)*
A roasting pan for roasting vegetables (CorningWare is fine too)	
	A set of glass storage containers

Note: Please do not buy Teflon-coated or nonstick pots and pans. Teflon and other nonstick coatings contain chemicals such as PFOA, linked to birth defects in animals. Buy enameled or porcelain-coated cast iron or stainless steel–lined because unlined copper and aluminum can dissolve into the food.

Some Final Thoughts Before We Begin

Congratulations. By preparing your kitchen, you have tackled the biggest Daily Beat in the book.

Although it may not feel like it, turning your kitchen inside out is a major healing act. You are already moving back to a more natural way of eating. And to some degree, you are no longer buying into the profoundly unhealthy yet socially accepted foods of our modern times.

One of my favorite thinkers and philosophers, Jiddu Krishnamurti, said, "It is no measure of health to be well adjusted to a profoundly sick society."

I completely agree. I think that people like you who are Spent are actually the healthier people. Your bodies are saying, "*No. I will not adjust to something that is this deeply unhealthy—as much as you try.*" In a way, I believe that Spent is the natural rhythm of our bodies resisting the unnatural rhythms we keep trying to impose upon them. Spent is the body's way of fighting and asking you to slow down and listen to it. In my mind, this means that if you are Spent, you have a natural rhythm that is strong enough to revolt and that is just waiting for you to give it the opportunity to thrive. So let's begin moving you back to the beat nature intended for you—your body is waiting!

PART II

Six Weeks of Healing:
The Spent Restorative Program

Week 1

Nourish

The real voyage of discovery lies not in seeking new lands, but in seeing with new eyes.

—Marcel Proust

The first week of the Spent restorative program is devoted to nourishing your depleted body. If you are anything like most of my Spent patients, for months—maybe even years—you have been operating on a sorry diet, poor sleep, and not enough downtime. If you were a plant, you'd be the withered one in the dark corner. Your body is hungry. For real food. For rest. For relaxation.

Week one is seven days of gentle revival. As with any plant, we don't want to shock your body with too much change.

We will take out two major Spent-causing food substances: sugars and processed foods. And we will begin bringing you back to life with nutritious smoothies, some tension-releasing physical stretches, and a few breathing exercises that will relax your body and ease your mind.

By day seven, you will already have more energy, better focus, and less pain.

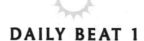

DAILY BEAT 1

CREATE A SWEETER LIFE

White sugar and artificial sweeteners are corrosive to everyone's health and well-being, but for those of us who are already stressed and tired, they are poison. White sugar disrupts key physiological systems, putting the body on a roller coaster of unnatural and extremely taxing highs and lows that make us feel Spent. And artificial sweeteners trick the body into over-eating and have toxic side effects.[1]

Your body processes sugar rapidly. As you know, when you eat sugars you get an initial burst of energy—the sugar hits your bloodstream almost as quickly as if you had mainlined it. Overwhelmed by the surge of sugar, the body scrambles to process it, producing insulin to transport the sugar from the bloodstream into the cells. This increase in insulin makes your blood sugar level drop. So the energy surge vanishes almost as quickly as it arrived and you "crash." This process triggers the body to crave more energy. So you eat more sugar or sugary carbohydrates to get the energy high again. A vicious cycle of craving, eating, and crashing begins.

Overwhelming the body with sugar daily puts enormous stress on your hormones. When you crash, your adrenal glands need to kick in and release cortisol, a steroidlike substance, to help lift you back up. Over time, your adrenal glands exhaust themselves trying to regulate your fluctuating sugar levels. This constant process of adjusting and rebalancing ultimately makes you feel exhausted.

An excess of cortisol in your system is also linked to weight gain. What's more, too much cortisol at the wrong times can initiate an inflammatory process that researchers now believe triggers chronic diseases, including diabetes, arthritis, allergies, some forms of cancer—and, I believe, Spent.

There has been some amazing research in the last few years about the effect of sugar on the body. Not only does eating too much sugar lead to obesity, diabetes, and tooth decay, it is also one of the biggest contributors to low energy and feelings of being overwhelmed—it has even been scientifically linked to depression.

Sugars are also admittedly one of the most difficult substances (notice I don't call them foods) for most people to take out of their diet. If you are still thinking, "There's no way I can do this," here are some more scary facts from Nancy Appleton's *Lick the Sugar Habit* for added motivation and inspiration:

- *Sugar can suppress the immune system.*
- *Sugar feeds cancer cells and has been linked to breast, ovarian, prostate, and rectal cancer.*
- *Sugar can weaken eyesight and cause premature skin aging.*
- *Sugar can cause premature aging in general and increase your risk of Alzheimer's disease.*
- *Sugar can cause autoimmune diseases, arthritis, asthma, heart disease, migraines, and multiple sclerosis.*[2]

To heal from Spent, you *must* cut sugars not only out of your kitchen but also out of your diet as much as possible.

As a fellow former sugar junkie (believe me, I feel your pain), I'm very sorry to say this means NOT EATING the following versions or anything with these versions or varieties of sugar in any of your food: brown sugar, fructose, sucrose, glucose, maltose, succinate, molasses, date sugar, beet sugar, grape sugar, cane sugar, corn syrup, high-fructose corn syrup, corn sugar, fruit juice concentrate, sorbitol, barley malt, caramel, carob syrup, maltodextrin, dextran, dextrose, sorghum syrup.

Unfortunately, as you learned in the Prepare section, it's not a great idea to replace sugar with artificial sweeteners. Though artificial sweeteners don't necessarily trigger the same kind of harmful hormonal cascade as white and processed sugars do, the chemicals in them are equally harmful. For instance, aspartame (the generic name of NutraSweet and Equal) is a dangerous food additive that some studies have shown has toxic effects, including triggering or worsening epilepsy, Parkinson's disease, and brain tumors. And though Splenda claims to be made from sugar, it is made by chlorinating sugar. This means if you use Splenda, you are essentially dumping chlorine into your coffee. As I will discuss later, chlorine is one of the harmful chemicals that most of us come into contact with on a daily basis. See www.sweetpoison.com for more information. For now, you must take these artificial sweeteners out: aspartame (NutraSweet and Equal), saccharin (Sweet'N Low), sucralose (Splenda), acesulfame K.

No sugars or artificial sweeteners means *not drinking* sodas, diet sodas, or fruit juice (unless freshly squeezed) and *not eating* candy, cakes, cookies, ice cream, most factory-made breads, many crackers and breakfast cereals, condiments such as ketchup, and salad dressings. Because sugars are so prevalent in our food, I could go on for pages. Suffice it to say that you must read food labels carefully, looking for the offending names I just listed. Please remember, when reading labels, that 4 grams of sugar is equivalent to 1 teaspoon.

My take on sugars may seem a little extreme to you, but my opinion is informed by my more than a quarter century of clinical experience with people who are Spent. As I see it, sugar is a socially acceptable, legal recreational drug. Like other recreational drugs, sugar can lead to mood highs and lows. And like other drugs, sugar can destroy your health over time and lead to Spent. Most people I see in my practice are sugar addicts—their behavior and emotions are somewhat controlled by sugar, even though they don't realize it and would probably deny it if I suggested it.

Just take a look at how addicted we Americans have become to the white crystalline substance. Most people use sugar in their coffee and have either bagels, pancakes, cereal, muffins, or fruit-flavored yogurt to get going in the morning, all of which contain lots of sugar. Then, for lunch, it's soda, ketchup, sugar-laden processed bread, and salad covered with a dressing that is also usually loaded with sugar. Then there's the addition of wine and dessert at dinner, which is more sugar. In fact, sugar is such a major component of the typical American diet that we treat it like a food group. What's more, most of the "complex" carbohydrates we consume, even those from so-called whole grains, including bagels and cereal, aren't really complex at all. They're often just as highly refined as foods made from white flour, and they act just like sugars in your body. We'll talk more about this in a few days. Remember, no matter what variety of sugar we are imbibing, apart from fruit, it is not a food. It is a high-calorie, nutritionally void, harmful substance.

I'd like to completely eliminate refined sugars from your diet, but I know how hard it was for me and many of my patients to get off sugar and find delicious alternatives. So I realize that it's unrealistic to expect you to go cold turkey. Although you probably won't experience withdrawal symptoms such as those experienced by, say, a heroin junkie, you more than likely will suffer from headaches, moodiness, irritability, fatigue, and, in all probability, the uncontrollable desire for something sweet. So, as with any drug addiction, you have to have a flexible but structured plan to beat it.

If you came in to see me, I'd be able to assess your ability to wean yourself off sugar, and I'd adjust your withdrawal in a way appropriate for you; as I will note throughout this book, everyone is different, and what's right for one person may be wrong for another. As a reader, you need to make those determinations yourself. What's important is to maintain a healthy attitude, and to accept yourself and your progress with grace.

In my practice, when I tell patients to eliminate sugar, the two most common responses I get are from:

1. Those who tend to be perfectionists and are very hard on themselves. Not surprisingly, when they slip, it can be traumatic and upsetting.

2. Those who have a hard time seeing things through. These patients will quit and then, after a week or so, go on a sugar binge, feel awful, get back "on the wagon," quit in another week or so. This cycle of trying to get better and self-sabotaging will continue until they are in terrible shape and truly desperate for help.

As you well know, each of these tendencies, in its own way, can lead us to become Spent. So make a note of what your proclivity is: to take something too seriously or not to persevere. And make a decision now to try to approach and do this differently.

No matter what your tendency is, please know that it is common to initially have cravings when you stop eating sugar. Here's some advice about how to cope:

1. *Drink.* Lots of water (plain or sparkling) with fresh mint or a slice of lemon or lime.

2. *Eat.* When you eliminate sugars, which, for many, are a major component of the daily diet, it is important to replace them with something nourishing. All week, I will offer you suggestions for how to incorporate alternatives—breakfast smoothies that are sweet, delicious, and chock-full of good nutrients, healthy snacks to replace the old nibble foods, and so on. But I would also suggest that you load up on the Spent Superfoods—the more nourishing your meals are, the less you will need the energy "boost" that you once got from sugar. And remember that a craving for "sugar" may actually just be a signal that you are hungry. So take a few deep breaths and then make the choice to put something nourishing in your mouth—a colorful salad, some nuts, or even a piece of chicken or fish. And if you need something sweet, have a piece of fruit. A great option is an ounce of 70% or 85% dark chocolate or any one of the breakfast smoothies or desserts in the Recipes for Renewal section in the back of the book. If these don't work, try a cup of organic plain yogurt with a touch of stevia or a teaspoon of raw honey or agave syrup.

3. *Take glutamine,* 1,000 milligrams every 4 to 6 hours, as necessary on an empty stomach, as it is an amino acid and may not be absorbed as well if taken with protein. This supplement tricks the brain into thinking it is getting glucose and therefore lowers sugar cravings. If the sugar cravings are bad, you can take 500 milligrams every hour. Glutamine is benign and has no side effects. In fact, it has been shown to boost the immune system and is an essential nutrient for the intestines. Occasionally, I have seen very large doses of glutamine cause an upset stomach, but this is very rare and occurs at much higher doses than I am recommending. For more information on glutamine, go to www.spentmd.com.

4. If you must have something sweet in your coffee or tea, then use small amounts of these healthy alternatives: stevia, agave, or

xylitol (which are the best options). The second best options are unprocessed raw honey or 100% pure organic maple syrup.

As the days go by (no, you are not giving up sugar for just one day), take it easy and do the best you can. If you find yourself scarfing down a brownie, don't let the slip add to your stress. It's no failure to fall off the wagon. I want to encourage you to adopt a healthy lifestyle, a healthy way of eating that you can sustain over time. Rather than making you feel so deprived that you react by sinking into a destructive sugar binge, I'd much rather you allow yourself something small and sweet every now and then— maybe have a small treat every fifth day.

Finally, while I realize that not eating sugars is perhaps the most excruciating thing I could ask you to do, just try it. After three or four days without sugars, you will feel much lighter and less Spent. And although this is just the beginning, please know that once you conquer your sugar addiction, it's all downhill from here.

As I mentioned in the introduction, I will be finishing each Daily Beat with what I'm calling "The Pulse." I've created this section to help you establish and stay in touch with your new rhythm. "The Pulse" section illustrates how to put each day's beat into action. "The Pulse" section also serves as a reminder, helping you keep track of things such as not eating sugar or artificial sweeteners, which you will be trying for the next few weeks.

I will remind you of a new suggestion for a few days and then give you the opportunity to try to integrate this new habit or dietary change into your life on your own. Then, after a few days or a week, we will revisit it. New suggestions are in bold type and marked with a ●; repeated suggestions are indicated with a ○. It has been my experience that sometimes my patients need and want these reminders and sometimes they don't. But, generally speaking, almost everyone on the program (including me) has had a day where he or she has thought, "I know I am forgetting to do something." Or "I could really use a push to do this." I hope these beats will be that wanted reminder or push.

The Pulse

○ ● ● ○ ● ● ○ ● ● ○

- Begin the Spent restorative eating program by eliminating sugars and artificial sweeteners from your diet. If you have a major craving for a sweet treat or snack in the afternoon or after dinner, get up from wherever you are sitting, walk around, drink a glass of water, and have a piece of fruit.
- If you haven't already bought glutamine, a powdered greens product and a whey protein product, then go to your local health food market or www.spentmd.com, which has my favorite recommendations on these products. I will explain how to use them tomorrow.
- Begin taking 1,000 milligrams of glutamine every 4 to 6 hours, as necessary.
- Buy a can of tennis balls. You will need them soon.

DAILY BEAT 2

REINVENT BREAKFAST

When stopping refined sugars and artificial sweeteners, breakfast is the meal that poses the biggest challenge, because no sugar means no pancakes, French toast, bagels, muffins, most cereals, or toast (any factory-made bread contains sugar). Breakfasts like these are not only nutritionally disastrous, they couldn't be worse for helping your body reestablish its natural rhythm. And, as you are learning, returning to your natural rhythm is essential for healing Spent.

A breakfast that heals Spent is one that is full of protein and good fats, in addition to some carbohydrates. Though eggs or plain organic yogurt are better options than cereal or bagels, they are not very exciting and not the best thing to be eating all the time. Personally, after a few days of plain yogurt or boiled eggs, my taste buds are bored. Knowing this, I've tried to provide you with options that are flexible, tasty, and satisfying—and will accommodate your morning routine. A full list of recipes and options is in the recipe section in the back of the book (page 268), but I believe a breakfast smoothie is the perfect rhythm-restoring, nutritious, delicious, and efficient way to begin your day. My patients continually tell me how they go to sleep at night dreaming of their breakfast smoothies. They are also invaluable because of the variety. They can be made in nearly endless combinations, which is important—some days our bodies need more fruit, and some days we need to include a heavier dose of protein.

I have a smoothie every morning. This quick, easy breakfast gives me the protein and good fats needed to start my day. Smoothies are also easy on my digestive system, as the body does not need to work to break down the food and nutrients. Digestion takes up a lot of energy, and by partially resting it, I am able to save on sorely needed energy that can be used else-where. When you are Spent, having more energy available is a good thing.

Each week, I will be suggesting a smoothie of the week that is spe-cially designed to support the dietary focus. This week, try one or two of my favorite basic smoothies, the Banana Berry Smoothie or the Blueberry Avocado Smoothie. But if these don't appeal to your palate or you don't have a lot of time in the morning, try my Workday Wonder Smoothie or another one from the recipe section.

Note: While not a thick smoothie, the Workday Wonder Smoothie provides all the essential nutrients for a complete breakfast. It can also be made at work since the ingredients are in powdered forms, eliminating the "I don't have time for breakfast" excuse.

Part of getting the body back into rhythm is learning to listen to ourselves—what we are really craving and what feels good. So, if you have already checked out the recipes and the Greeno Mojito Avocado Smoothie sounds better . . . even amazing (which it is), whip it up!

Avocados may not seem like a natural breakfast food or, for that matter, a smoothie ingredient, but my wife, Janice, and I discovered that they bring the most incredible texture to our smoothies, making them as creamy as milk shakes or puddings. Replacing bananas with avocados decreases the sugar content and adds good fats. Avocados are loaded with good fats and magnesium, both of which are much needed when you are Spent. Because of this, avocados are my preferred base ingredient for breakfast smoothies. A deficiency of magnesium is common when you are Spent and can lead to muscle pain, headaches, constipation, fatigue, and insomnia.

The other smoothie ingredient that I am a big fan of is whey protein. I use and suggest all my patients use whey protein in their morning shake because whey is an easy-to-digest protein. More important, it contains all the essential amino acids; in particular, cysteine, which is a precursor to glutathione, which decreases as you age. Glutathione is essential in your body's detoxification processes, boosts the immune system, and is one of the most important antioxidants in your body. Make sure the whey you buy comes from cows that grazed on pesticide- and chemical-free grass and were never fed grain or given growth hormones, chemicals, or antibiotics.

And, in all of my smoothie recipes, except the chocolate avocado one (which is an incredible treat!), I suggest that you add a super "greens" powder. Super greens powders will give you some of the essential vitamins and nutrients you need to heal Spent. Go to www.spentmd.com for all my favorite products.

A recent review conducted by the National Cancer Institute found that a staggering 87 percent of American families do not get the minimum recommended amount of fruits and vegetables (five to nine servings a day) required to maintain health.[3,4] A cup of raw vegetables or fruit or half a cup of cooked vegetables constitutes one serving. This finding supports the conclusion by many experts that the current American diet has already led to increased incidents of nutrient deficiencies, obesity, and chronic diseases.

Traditional vitamin supplements cannot make up for this dietary deficiency. They do not have the variety of fruits, vegetables, and grasses, so rich in vitamins, minerals, and the phytochemicals—the key ingredients in fruits and vegetables—that are essential generally to health and well-being and specifically to treating Spent. Greens powders come the closest to supplying these essential nutrients.

Although I recommend eating fruits and vegetables, greens drinks have inherent advantages over certain fruits and some vegetables (such as carrots, which can elevate one's blood sugar levels excessively if eaten in large quantities). Because greens drinks contain only the extract of the pigments—where the nutrients are highly concentrated—they are a superior way to derive the essence of fruits and vegetables without consuming the excess sugars and calories. Moreover, as with smoothies, rather than asking the body to work to digest a plate of kale or bowl of broccoli, the body can process and absorb the greens drink nutrients easily. Again, less digestive work means more energy.

I cannot think of a better breakfast food than a smoothie with greens in it. I am so convinced of a smoothie's healing potential for those who are Spent that if changing your diet to eat a smoothie every morning were the only thing you took away from this book and integrated into your life, I would be satisfied.

As I mentioned in the Prepare chapter, as we take empty foods out, I like to replace them with natural nutrients and pure foods. As we go through this process, you'll note that I always stipulate that foods preferably be organic, whole, filtered, and unprocessed. This is because I believe the quality of the foods we eat is critical.

Final note: Although whey protein comes from dairy, most people, even those sensitive to dairy, tolerate it well. Occasionally I have seen patients get gas and bloating from whey. If this happens, switch to a powder with rice protein.

The Pulse

○ ● ● ○ ● ● ○ ● ● ○

- **Try making a Banana Berry, Blueberry Avocado, or Workday Wonder Smoothie.**
- ○ Continue to follow the Spent restorative eating program, liberating your body from sugar and artificial sweeteners. Know that the first three days without sugar are the worst. At the end of the day, you will be two thirds of the way through!
- ○ Continue taking 1,000 milligrams of glutamine every 4 to 6 hours, as necessary.

SLEEP BEAT

For the last two days, we have focused on your diet, but, as I said in my introduction, Spent is multifaceted and therefore must be treated on many levels. Tonight we will begin what will be an ongoing discussion of your sleep habits. All the Sleep Beats are about teaching you how to better relax and release your mind and body to prepare for sleep. Most of us come home from a day of work feeling exhausted yet completely wound up from too much stimulation. The sleep and release techniques I will be teaching you will help soothe your mind and body, allowing your body to make a better vertical to horizontal transition. The first rule for better sleeping is:

Don't watch TV in bed.

There are only two things you should do in bed, and they both begin with the letter "S," as in sleep and sex. Save other activities, such as watching TV, working on your laptop, knitting, or even reading, for your easy chair. Though some of my patients tell me that watching TV or reading in bed helps them fall asleep, I generally don't recommend it.

Many of us are photosensitive. Yes, like the leaves on trees. The light from watching television or working at the computer may prevent our sleeping rhythm from kicking in. In particular, the bright light of a TV or computer may stop our melatonin levels from rising to induce sleep because our body still thinks it is daytime. You may think of the hormone melatonin simply as an over-the-counter sleep supplement, but it is much more than this. In terms of the body's overall rhythm and health, it plays a key role. Melatonin induces sleep and helps regulate our body's circadian rhythm, synchronizing our internal body clock. When you are Spent, your body clock is off. Melatonin is also a strong and versatile antioxidant. It boosts the immune system, and some studies show that it can even fight aging.

All this is to say that if you watch TV after 10 p.m., you are more than likely interrupting your body's natural rhythm and need to slow down and sleep. If you have a show you must watch, these days it is easy enough to record it.

Special note on melatonin: As a supplement, melatonin can be helpful if you have trouble falling asleep, but it does not serve those who suffer from waking up frequently or too early, as it stays in the system for only an hour. A small dose of .5 milligram can be helpful to some people. If it doesn't work after a week, you can increase the dose to 1 milligram for another three weeks. If it still hasn't helped, I don't recommend upping the dose or continuing to use it, as there are no studies on the effects of long-term use—and it might interrupt the body's own production of melatonin. Finally, I don't recommend melatonin for anyone under forty, as your system already has enough.

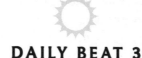

DAILY BEAT 3

PRACTICE THE ULTIMATE NECK
AND SHOULDER RELEASE

One of the major complaints I hear from new patients who are Spent is that they have an achy body. They carry tension and have pain in their shoulders or lower backs and have generally tired, sore muscles and joints. They have almost always seen other doctors before they come to see me. They've been given steroid shots and anti-inflammatory drugs, have been told they are just "getting old," and in some cases surgery has been recommended or even performed. Not one of these solutions treats the most common cause: tight and dysfunctional fascia.

I'll bet that in all the visits you've ever made to your doctor, the word "fascia" has never once been mentioned. And I'm not surprised, because for reasons unknown to me, this "organ" is largely ignored by Western medicine. It's shocking, when you think of it, that most doctors never address this thin, tough membrane that surrounds and is fused with your bones, muscles, tendons, nerves, blood vessels, and organs throughout your body. It is the organ that literally connects you from head to toe. The fascia helps muscles change shape and lengthen during movement and allows them to move easily over one another. It also aids in the repair of injuries and provides pathways for nerves, blood, and lymphatic vessels. It is involved in all aspects of motion and enhances your posture.

I explain to my patients that chronic musculoskeletal pain is frequently due to tight, constricted fascia, which occurs when the body compensates for an untreated or improperly treated injury. Contrary to what we have been conditioned to believe, pain is not a natural outcome of the aging process. As a matter of fact, chronic musculoskeletal pain is usually preventable and even reversible. I explain that by releasing the tightness in their fascia and tension in their muscles, they will have immediate relief and healing.

In Western medicine, we excel at treating acute trauma such as broken bones and torn cartilage, but we're pretty clueless when it comes to treating soft-tissue injuries. Soft tissues are your muscles and connective tissues, which include tendons, ligaments, and your body's forgotten stepchild, the fascia.

The most common problems any primary care doctor sees are sprains, muscle strains, and neck and low back pain problems—most of which are soft-tissue injuries in which the fascia is almost always a factor. Most doctors consider these to be minor, self-limiting problems, since they're not life-threatening, and assume that the pain will eventually go away. Instead of treating the soft tissues involved (muscles, tendons, ligaments, and, most important, the fascia), doctors tend to give anti-inflammatory drugs or shoot steroids into a stiff or sore area. The steroids temporarily alleviate the pain by reducing inflammation, but neither the drugs nor the injections address the underlying problem. As a result, other pains, knots, and constrictions develop in the fascia. Since the fascia is one continuous system running throughout the body, a tightening in one area also affects other areas. That's why an inappropriately treated sprained ankle, for instance, can morph into chronic pain elsewhere in the body and can eventually lead to generalized, chronic inflammation.

Let me explain how a soft-tissue injury, such as a sprain or strain, can become the "pebble in the pond" whose ripple effect can wreak painful havoc throughout your body. Just think of what happens to your body when you limp from a sore ankle: the muscles and other tissues on the opposite side of your body from the injury move in unnatural ways to help support the extra weight that's not being placed on the sore side. Then the "healthy" side becomes stressed and you start having a sore knee or hip on that side—and before you know it, that hurt ankle has traveled up your body so that you now have a sore ankle on one side, a stiff knee or hip on the other, and a tight shoulder and back on the hurt ankle side that is trying to compensate for the stiffness in the knee or hip—and then it spirals up to your neck. And then you are basically hurting all over.

If you treat the soft tissues that hurt and restore the proper functioning of the soft tissues involved (usually muscles, but also the fascia, tendons, and ligaments), your body will heal *without overstressing itself elsewhere.*

Having a pain-free body is a key component of wellness. As you know, if your body hurts, it tires you out and even interrupts the sleep you so desperately need when you are Spent. So tonight, spend a little time playing with one of my favorite fascia releases, using two tennis balls. Most of my patients call it "The Ultimate Neck and Shoulder Release." I guarantee that your neck and shoulders will not be the same after this.

The Pulse
○ • • ○ • • ○ • • ○

○   Start your day with another breakfast smoothie.

•   If you haven't already done so, buy a can of tennis balls today so that you can try the release at home tonight.

•   Order a foam roller today. In the coming days, I'll be teaching you other fascia release exercises, including a few techniques that use a foam roller. A foam roller is one of my favorite tools to use to help the body move back into balance and release the fascia. And, for around $15.00, you can't get a cheaper back massage or adjustment! I like the ones offered by Exertools (www.exertools.com)—they are a bit higher in density than other versions on the market.

○   Continue to follow the Spent restorative eating program, liberating your body from sugar and artificial sweeteners.

○   Continue taking 1,000 milligrams of glutamine every 4 to 6 hours, as necessary.

SLEEP BEAT

○   Don't forget to turn your TV off by 10 p.m.!

•   Try the Ultimate Neck and Shoulder Release before bed. As I said yesterday, most of us do not pay enough attention to getting ourselves ready for bed. Unwinding and relaxing tense muscles is one of the best ways to help the body transition from racing around to restoring itself. Play with this for a few minutes before you crawl into bed. It works wonders.

ULTIMATE NECK AND SHOULDER RELEASE

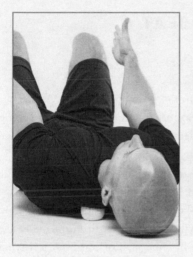 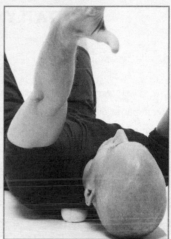

Lie on your back, knees bent and feet hip width apart so that your kneecaps are in line with your hip bones. Place two tennis balls at the top of your shoulder blades, side by side, in the area where you would love to have a massage. Slowly lower your head and shoulders. Place a pillow behind your head if your neck is uncomfortable. Lift your arms to the ceiling, then move them slowly toward your knees and then toward the wall behind you. Repeat this 10 times. To get even better results, pause on the tender areas for at least 10 seconds.

*   ***Option (not shown):*** *Open your arms toward the sides of the room into a "T" position, then return them over your chest. Repeat 10 times.*

*   ***Benefits:*** *Releases tight upper back, neck, and shoulder muscles. Can help with neck pain, headaches, shoulder concerns, and often even elbow and wrist issues related to tight fascia in the neck and shoulder area as well as loss of shoulder mobility.*

*   ***Caution:*** *Avoid placing tennis balls under your neck.*

*   ***Special note about the release techniques:*** *If this or any of the other release techniques I teach you feels good and you want to integrate it into your daily routine for a while, by all means, go ahead. Remember: releasing stress from the body is a great way to prepare for sleep!*

DAILY BEAT 4

If your particular flavor of Spent leans more toward mental stress, anxiety, or even panic attacks, today's beat will offer some relief. This breathing technique helps every one of my patients ease tension and adopt a steadier, less racy rhythm throughout their busy days. So don't skip this beat!

My patient Patti was recruited (along with her friend and college roommate Isobel) by a hedge fund at three times her previous salary. Though she loved the job initially, she soon began feeling tired, anxious, and depressed, and she couldn't sleep properly. For the first time in her life, she started having panic attacks—tight chest, loss of breath. A terrifying experience for anyone.

Meanwhile, her friend Isobel was thriving. Though she experienced the same on-the-job stress as Patti did, it didn't seem to affect her. Patti told me that Isobel loved her job but also had the ability to see her job as just a job. On the other hand, Patti, who was single with no family close by, worked as though her job were her life.

Patti decided to buy an apartment. She had visions that it would serve as a sanctuary from work. But it completely backfired. Now, with a hefty mortgage, she felt even more at the mercy of her job, fearing being fired. In short, her new, fabulous six-figure salary did nothing but bring more anxiety and stress into Patti's life.

Finally, Patti came to me, desperate for relief. I insisted that she follow the complete Spent restorative eating program, adding supplements and my adaptogenic formula (which you will learn about soon) to support her healing. But the key piece of her recovery was teaching her to use her breath to relax and restore her energy.

I told Patti to pay attention when her mind began to run on a hamster wheel of worry. As soon as she felt herself moving into a spiral of negative thinking, I asked her to push back from her desk, place both feet flat on the floor, lay her hands in her lap, close her eyes, and take three minutes to feel her feet touching the floor and reconnect with her breathing—noticing that she was breathing in; noticing that she was breathing out.

This simple exercise of getting out of her head, feeling her feet, and sensing herself inhale and exhale served as an amazing tool for Patti. Observing her breath move in and out helped her relieve the oppressive stress she felt at work. By grounding herself and interrupting her negative thought patterns, she had more energy and creativity for her work and life. In fact, Patti found meditating on the breath so helpful that, on her next vacation, she took off for a ten-day mindfulness retreat!

As we all know, the problems, situations, and people we encounter on a daily basis don't necessarily cause us nearly as much stress as our *reaction* to them does. It's all about how we perceive our world. Patti internalized her stress in a way that made her sick, while her friend Isobel, exposed to the very same stress, was able to deflect it.

Quieting and slowing our breath stimulate what is called the parasympathetic response, which calms the body down—the perfect antidote to the overstressed state we are in.

I can't tell you how many times I've felt tension rising in my body and I've gone into my office, closed the door, sat down, visualized putting my energy into my feet, connecting with the floor, and watched my breath, imagining the inhale moving all the way down to my toes and the exhale moving from my soles to my shoulders. Five minutes later, I walk out to treat patients feeling like a new man.

BREATHING FOR MINDFULNESS AND RELAXATION

Read through the following instructions a few times and then try this. Don't worry about memorizing exactly how to do it. There is no right or wrong way. This is just to give you an idea or sense of how to breathe mindfully to relax.

Sit in a chair, preferably one with a straight back. Place both feet flat on the floor, and lay your hands in your lap or gently on top of your thighs. You can close your eyes or leave them open, but many people find closing their eyes easier because there are fewer distractions. Begin by bringing your energy down to your feet and feeling the floor as you "watch" your inhale and exhale with your mind. Breathe in through your nose, allowing the breath to move into the back of your body and down to your feet. Exhale through your nose, allowing the breath to soften the front of your body—easing the thighs, ribs, and shoulders. When you notice your mind wandering, just come back to your feet and breath. It is completely normal to lose your focus on your breath to an interesting thought or idea, so when you notice you have lost your focus, gently bring your attention back to your inhale and exhale. Don't force or control the breath. Simply inhale through the nose and exhale through the nose. Easy soft breaths. Inhaling and exhaling.

If you feel uncomfortable doing this at your desk or in a room with family or friends and want privacy, you can simply go to the bathroom, put the lid down on the toilet, and sit there. You can also move to another free space for a moment. Or, if it is nice outside, find a bench or a tree to sit under. But don't make finding the space a big production. This is about finding and making space for you, bringing your attention back to your breath, and quietly listening to your body's natural rhythm. Another great alternative is the One Global Breath meditation tool at www.spentmd .com.

The Pulse
○ • • ○ • • ○ • • ○

○ Continue to follow the Spent restorative eating program, liberating your body from sugar and artificial sweeteners.

○ Continue taking 1,000 milligrams of glutamine every 4 to 6 hours, as necessary.

○ Have a protein- and phytonutrient-rich breakfast today—preferably a smoothie.

● **Throughout the day, take a few mini–breathing breaks to help fight your sugar cravings and stress.**

SLEEP BEAT

Two nights ago, I talked about how watching TV can throw your mela-tonin production off. Your cell phone and computer can also throw your body off. There is an ever growing debate about how the electromagnetic frequencies (EMFs) from cell phones and wireless computers affect our health. There is enough evidence now to at least put a little "caution" sticker on them in our minds. Think how tired your mind, eyes, and ears are after a long session on a cell phone or computer. That's really all the evidence you need to know that these devices drain your energy. Since many of us spend most of our days with our cell phones glued to our heads and/or our heads bent over a wirelessly connected computer, I think it is worth trying to decrease this potentially dangerous exposure as much as we can. Let's give our bodies a rest at night when we sleep—especially if these devices are in our bedroom!

- Turn your TV off at 10 p.m. or earlier, and at the same time, turn off your cell phones, handheld devices like Blackberrys, iPhones, and Treos, wireless connections, and computers. If you must keep them on, keep them as far away from your head as possible.

DAILY BEAT 5

UNPROCESS YOUR DIET

Like sugar, processed fats and processed foods are toxic to the body—particularly for those who are Spent. When I talk about processing, I am talking about the practice of taking valuable food and physically altering it by heating it, refining it, and adding sugars, salt, artificial colors, and preservatives to add taste and texture and increase shelf life. This "process" transforms that original food into a substance that has far less nutritional value and far more things that are bad for you.

As you have probably gathered, my philosophy is: nature has done just fine, giving us a plethora of extraordinary and delicious foods, so why mess with it? The best example of just how we can make a good thing bad is illustrated by hydrogenation.

Hydrogenation is a process that changes liquid, unsaturated, relatively healthy oil into a more solid form, which increases a product's shelf life and helps make foods with a smoother texture. When the fat becomes solid, the body treats it more like a saturated fat, although it is not classified as saturated fat on food labels. But hydrogenation has serious health consequences because it creates trans fats. Trans fats are polyunsaturated vegetable oils that have been processed to make them remain solid at room temperature. Trans fats also come from frying food in polyunsaturated vegetable oils, such as corn oil, sunflower oil, safflower oil, and soy oil, all of which are not bad for you until they are heated.

As you may know, trans fats increase the level of bad LDL cholesterol in your bloodstream and lower your level of good HDL cholesterol. According to Dr. Walter Willett, professor of nutrition and epidemiology at the Harvard School of Public Health, trans fats in food cause at least 30,000 premature deaths in the United States each year.[5]

But trans fats are really bad for people with Spent because, when you eat trans fats, they block the uptake and use of good essential fatty acids, such as omega-3s, omega-6s, and omega-9s, which people who are Spent desperately need. Essential fatty acids are crucial to healthy brain function, healthy eyes, joints, skin, and hair, as well as our immune system. They reduce inflammation and the risk of heart disease. Among other things, they help create elastic cell membranes. When the body doesn't have these healthy fats, it turns to the unhealthy fats to build cell membranes. As you can imagine, cell membranes made with unhealthy fats are not quite up to par. Trans fats not only disrupt healthy cell function but also become poor building blocks that result in a more fragile system.

Likewise, chemically processed foods and foods that include preservatives and flavor enhancers make our cells work very hard and weaken the body. Because these chemicals are not derived from nature, our genes have no program for processing them. The body—particularly the immune system—greets these foreign substances like aliens, attacking them and flushing them out. Though these chemicals may make your food a pretty color or longer-lasting, they sap your energy, exhaust your immune system, and weaken your body.

This is why, for the next few weeks (and hopefully forever), I'd like you to stop eating processed foods and anything containing hydrogenated fats or oils. As with sugar, these foods bring us nothing but fatigue and weakness, which is exactly what we are trying to avoid.

Depending upon your current diet, my list of the processed foods to cut may freak you out or not. Please know that, as with sugar, I don't expect you to change everything in one day. More than likely, you'd be even more Spent if you did try to go directly from loads of processed foods to none. But I want no processed foods and fats to be a *goal* that you can work toward over the course of the next few weeks. This is why I am offering you a fairly complete list of processed foods. As you begin to feel better and embrace this process, you will have a helpful and thorough reference.

Not eating refined or processed foods means not eating:

White rice
All quick-cooking rice, including quick-cooking brown rice
Any refined grain such as farina, quick oats, or boxed side dishes with processed grains; so
   no parmesan couscous, wild rice dishes, or anything else that says "quick" or "easy"
Factory-made breads—this means most breads on the supermarket shelves
Bagels (which are usually loaded with sugar as well)

Commercial breakfast cereals (including instant oats)

Cakes, cupcakes, pies, doughnuts, and pastries (just a reminder; you should have cut these out when you stopped sugar)

Crackers and pretzels

Chips (all kinds—even organic corn or soy chips)

Processed cheeses such as American, Velveeta, cream cheese, etc.

Frozen meals

Most packaged snack foods—for example, anything in a "single-serving" package— from candy bars to "health" bars like Luna Bars, Power Bars, and Clif Bars

Fried food—this means no fast food, no French fries, no home fries, no fried chicken, and so on

Processed meats—this includes hot dogs, salami, sausage, ham, bacon, deli meats, and other packaged lunch meats

Margarine

Though challenging at first, eliminating all processed, refined, and junk food from your diet is one of the most powerful actions you can take to heal from Spent. Tomorrow I will give you some tips on how to eat and survive without these old "staples." But if you are looking for some delicious replacements for today, check out the Snack Attack section on page 301, or go to www.spentmd.com for more options.

The Pulse
○ • • ○ • • ○ • • ○

○ Have a smoothie for breakfast.

● **Make a concerted effort to free your diet of processed foods and foods with hydrogenated or partially hydrogenated fats or oils (trans fats).**

○ Continue to follow the Spent restorative eating program, liberating your body from sugar and artificial sweeteners.

○ Continue taking 1,000 milligrams of glutamine 4 four to 6 hours, as necessary.

SLEEP BEAT

- **Breathe mindfully before bed.**

If you have not found the time to try a breathing break or have tried it once but have not tried it again, before you go to bed, find a comfortable space, sit down, and spend five minutes or so watching your inhale and exhale. (For the full instructions, see pages 59 60.) If you have been trying the breathing breaks throughout your day and have found them helpful, try sitting for seven or ten minutes tonight right before you sleep. Watching the breath is a wonderful way to prepare for bed—it settles the mind, relaxes the body, and is a great way to transition out of your day.

○ Stop the overstimulation. Remember to turn off your TV, cell phones, and computers by 10 p.m.

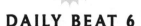

DAILY BEAT 6

FIND YOUR EATING RHYTHM

When it comes to having a healthy eating rhythm that supports our body's innate digestive functions and energy cycle, most of us make one or two of the following mistakes (though we are already working to correct the first one):

- *We don't eat enough of the right foods—particularly for breakfast— so our bodies are not nourished. We eat a carb-laden breakfast, and then we binge on sugary snack foods or caffeine in the late morning and afternoon to give ourselves a "boost."*
- *We fill ourselves up with nutrient-deficient food substances and then feel tired.*
- *We don't eat often enough, and then, when we are absolutely starving, we gorge ourselves.*
- *We eat our largest meal at dinner, when our digestive system is slowing down, instead of at lunch, when our digestion is at its peak.*

Throughout the next few weeks, I will be making suggestions to help you learn to listen to your body's food rhythms so that you can give your body the nutrients it needs at the right times. For instance, the first and very obvious suggestion is to *feed your body appropriately when it needs fuel.* Rather than having your biggest meal just before you go to sleep, when your body doesn't need to be charged up, eat a bigger breakfast and lunch, when digestion is at its peak, and have a smaller dinner. Eat small snacks to support your body in the late morning and afternoon.

In terms of our physiological food clock, soon after we wake up in the morning, our food clock signals us to have an appetite. It signals the liver and digestive system to process nutrients. By midday, the body's metabolism is reaching its peak. That is why breakfast and lunch should be your largest meals, because this is when your body is primed to deal with a lot of food. As daylight wanes, the body clock slows its secretion of the active daytime hormones and our metabolism slows down. For this reason you should not have a large meal at dinnertime. As Deborah Szekeley, the founder of the famous Rancho La Puerta Spa, says, "Make your salad plate your dinner plate and your dinner plate your salad plate." Making a large salad your main course for dinner is easy to do and makes a significant difference to the body's rhythms.

What you eat at what time of day does make a huge difference. The body needs proteins and fats in the morning (one of the reasons I suggested adding an avocado to your smoothie this week) for the activity and alertness needed during the day. It needs healthy carbohydrates at night for the relaxation and detoxification functions that occur while we sleep.

A few days ago, I encouraged you to eat a protein- and nutrient-rich breakfast, which, for me, is my first beat in the rhythm of eating. Having a good breakfast of appropriate foods sets the day's rhythm, so it is the most important. But so is lunch, which we normally rush through. Making the shift to eating a bigger lunch and a smaller dinner is initially an effort, especially if you are inclined to have soup or a slice of pizza on the run for lunch and then a big dinner. But making lunch the largest meal makes an enormous difference and very often leads to weight loss (if desired).

The other way to keep your energy going throughout the day is to support the three meals—a protein-rich breakfast, a substantial lunch, when digestion is at its peak, and a smaller dinner—is by having two small snacks. Incorporating nutrient-rich snacks into our daily eating pattern is particularly helpful when we detox from sugar, processed fats and foods, and chemicals. Snacks ensure that we are nutritionally supported throughout the day and thus crave junk and unhealthy foods less.

As you know, I almost always start my day with a breakfast shake with protein, fat, and phytonutrients. I often don't feel hungry if I have a breakfast smoothie, but if I do, I snack on some nuts later in the morning. At around one, I have lunch, my biggest meal, consisting of protein and vegetables. Then, around four or five in the afternoon, I'll have a piece of fruit. Around seven, I'll have a smallish dinner that includes a small amount of protein, more vegetables, and healthy carbohydrates. By eating a nutritious breakfast with protein and good fats, a larger lunch, and a smaller dinner, *about the same time every day*, my body and its energy levels are regulated.

Having two small snacks, if necessary, means that I never get hungry or suffer from a sugar low. My body never has to be exhausted by searching for or expecting food, nor does it get tired out from the assault of a huge meal. It also has the nutrients it needs for both daytime and nighttime functioning.

Although timing what you eat is a powerful way to reestablish your body rhythms, finding a rhythm for eating is not just about what and when we eat, it also means rethinking *how* we eat. Fast food has done more than just make most of us Spent and addicted to unhealthy processed foods, sugar, and trans fats. It has also set a precedent and bred poor eating habits. We gulp our drinks and inhale our food while driving in our cars, while standing at counters, even while walking. It seems that we have completely lost the rite and ritual of sitting down at a table, chewing our food, and actually tasting it. Culinary-wise and socially, this is a great loss, but we also pay for it physically.

Most of us don't realize that digestion begins in the mouth. The process of chewing is an essential component of good digestion. The mechanical action of chewing breaks down large food molecules into smaller particles, and saliva contains enzymes that contribute to the chemical process of digestion. When food is not chewed well, bigger food particles pass through to the intestines, where they then become food for the trillions of bacteria in your gut. These larger particles can cause digestive symptoms and even overgrowth of the wrong bacteria in the intestines. The bigger the particles of food you give your stomach and intestines to break down, the more work they have to do. Over time, the digestive system gets tired of working so hard, and these big particles go into your bloodstream, where your immune system has to deal with them. Your immune system experiences the food as potentially toxic to your body, so it attacks the food and you can develop a reaction to that food. Sometimes giving your digestive system poorly chewed food can lead to what seems like an allergic response to a food that you are not necessarily allergic to.

But the benefits of chewing your food properly go well beyond improved digestion. Most important, it makes you slow down when you are eating. Food begins to taste better, you enjoy it more, and it can become almost like a meditation. Eating slowly means you are less likely to gain weight. When you eat too quickly, your brain doesn't have enough time to register the amount you've eaten or if it is enough, so it keeps asking for more. There is no mystery about what happens next: you gain weight.

Today I want you to begin to make a concerted effort to return to the table. To make your meals more than just a function of fueling your body. Here in this country we have such an extraordinary abundance of food that it is a crime not to celebrate our good fortune by enjoying the food on our tables. Honor your body by sitting down and slowing down to eat.

My guess is that you will find that eating in rhythm with your body's circadian rhythms will come naturally—because you are reflecting and feeding your biological needs! And, as you are, I hope, beginning to experience, when you get back to your natural rhythm, you get back to your more essential self, and Spent dissipates.

As I've mentioned before, in the back of this book—and at www .spentmd.com—there are dozens of recipes for salads and meals that are designed for this rhythm of eating, including my favorite snack recipes. One of my favorite snacks is Janice's trail mix, which I would encourage you to try today. The recipe is on page 301.

The Pulse
○ ● ● ○ ● ● ○ ● ● ○

- **Try playing with a new rhythm for eating today:**
  Have a protein-rich smoothie that includes healthy fats. Any of the smoothies is perfect for this! Midmorning, have a snack if you need to. Maybe try Janice's trail mix recipe on page 301. Make lunch, when your digestion is at its peak, your biggest meal. Have a salad with some protein. Sit down for lunch. Have a piece of fruit in the afternoon. For dinner, make your salad the main course and your main course the side plate. Add a healthy grain, like quinoa, brown rice, or brown rice pasta. Take your time and enjoy it. Notice if this new way of eating increases your energy level throughout the day.
- ○ Continue to follow the Spent restorative eating program,

liberating your body from sugar, artificial sweeteners, and processed foods.

○ Continue taking 1,000 milligrams of glutamine every 4 to 6 hours, as necessary.

○ Continue taking breathing breaks throughout the day. For instance, while at work, take three 3-minute breathing breaks.

SLEEP BEAT

○ Continue lowering your exposure to EMF by turning off your computer and cell phone. And continue not to confuse your circadian rhythms by watching TV late into the night.

● **Take a long bath to relax.** A bath is a wonderful and easy way to remove tension from and relax the muscles. Use Epsom salts—magnesium sulfate, which is absorbed by the skin, reduces inflammation and restores balance.

○ And if watching your breath helped prepare you for sleep last night, try it again!

DAILY BEAT 7

RESTORE YOURSELF

I am a huge fan of yoga and what it can do for the body. I have been practicing yoga for almost twenty years. I've seen a profound change in my body and the way I feel, not only physically but emotionally and psychologically too. But more impressive are the hundreds of patients I have seen over the years who have used yoga as a way to help them heal from Spent and move on to manage having very complex, stressful lives and still stay in rhythm.

I encourage you to invest some time and effort in finding a yoga class and establishing a yoga practice. But for our purposes, I will be giving you a few restorative yoga asanas (poses) in this book that are specifically designed for recovery from being Spent. These particular asanas have a profound healing effect on your body and mind.

Restorative yoga was developed by B. K. S. Iyengar, who has been teaching for more than sixty years and is universally recognized as an authority on yoga. Restorative yoga came about when he adapted yoga postures so that people who were incapacitated in some way could get the benefits from them without using up energy. Restorative yoga is particularly helpful when you feel run-down, burned out, stressed out, and Spent. It is also a powerful tool to help the healing process during and after an illness or injury. These are times when sleep, rest, and these supported poses are even more important, as energy must be conserved for the body to heal. I have found restorative yoga to be both healing and revitalizing, as one gets the effects of the poses without exerting any energy. You can imagine why a physical pose that is designed to restore the body is a profound tool for a person suffering from being Spent.

To do restorative yoga most effectively, you need props. These props help support the body and maintain the correct healing position without strain. This morning, I'll ask you to use a wall in your home to help you release your shoulders, hamstrings, and back. Tonight I will teach you a pose that requires just a blanket from around your house. But to really reap the benefits, it is best to invest in a few yoga props to help you and your body be properly (no pun intended) supported in the poses I will be teaching you in this book.

Try this restorative yoga pose before you head off to work:

WALL STRETCH

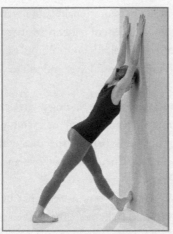

This opens the back of the legs and stretches the shoulders and syncs the body with the breath.

I chose this pose because nearly everyone can do it. Although it looks deceptively simple, when you do it, you'll find there is a lot going on. It is a great way to start the day as it affects the whole body very positively. It especially frees the shoulder joints. So work on it gradually if you have a shoulder problem or a very constricted shoulder girdle. It also releases tension in the hands, which these days are more overworked and tighter with everyone on their keyboards and BlackBerrys.

Begin by standing 3 to 4 feet away from a wall. Face the wall and place the ball of your left foot against it, with the foot bent at 45 degrees, as illustrated in the photo. Keep your weight on the center of your left heel and let your right foot turn out a little, as pictured.

Keep the front of your hips parallel to the wall and place your hands as far up the wall as you can reach. Open your hands, spreading your fingers, and straighten your elbows.

Keep your legs straight, firming your kneecaps onto the knee joint, and pull your thigh muscles up. Extend your back heel backward. Move your hips away from the wall while pressing the palms of your hands and your fingers into the wall. Let your neck relax and extend your head toward the wall. It may rest on the wall.

Stay in the pose for about 30 seconds, breathing normally. Then, keeping your hands on the wall, switch legs and practice the pose with your right foot against the wall and your left leg back. Make sure that your back foot is at about a 45-degree angle, with the heel firmly planted.

Special instructions:

1. *Open the fingers wide, pressing the knuckles of your index fingers against the wall. Keep your elbows straight and allow your shoulders to open as you move your hips away from the wall.*
2. *Remember to keep the front of your hips parallel to the wall as you perform these movements.*
3. *Most important, remember to breathe!*

The Pulse

○ ● ● ○ ● ● ○ ● ● ○

○   Continue to follow the Spent restorative eating program, liberating your body from sugar, artificial sweeteners, and processed foods.

○   If you are still having sugar cravings and find that glutamine is helping, then continue taking 1,000 milligrams of glutamine every 4 to 6 hours, as necessary. If your cravings have eased, you can stop.

○   Have another protein- and nutrient-rich breakfast, and don't forget to make lunch your biggest meal of the day.

○   Continue to take breathing breaks throughout the day. Watch your breath at lunch time.

●   Order a few yoga props:

· *One 10-foot belt, or strap. I prefer the D ring to the cinch strap. These belts cost about $8.00 to $12.00 each.*

· *Three yoga blankets. The cotton or acrylic "Mexican" ones are the cheapest. They cost about $24.00 apiece.*
· *A round bolster. Depending upon the materials, these cost from $50.00 to $80.00 and are well worth the expense.*
· *An eye mask. These cost about $12.00.*
· *A yoga mat, if you don't have one.*

The best place to purchase these props is on the Internet. The sites I've had the most success with are:

www.huggermugger.com

www.gaiam.com

www.yogaccessories.com

www.yogaprops.net

Note: I have found that a number of my patients are very reluctant to spend roughly $150.00 on yoga props. They think it is too much money to spend on something they don't really need or will never use. If you are in this camp, I understand. The reason I strongly recommend that you purchase yoga props is that a prop like a bolster helps you achieve more precise alignment and physical relaxation than a lumpy couch pillow does. If you don't feel like spending the money right now, that is fine. Try a few of the restorative yoga exercises using pillows, towels, and blankets from around your house, see if you like restorative yoga, and then make the decision whether to invest or not.

SLEEP BEAT

● To prepare for sleep tonight, I'd like you to try the basic Savasana (sha-*vah*-sah-na) or "corpse pose."

This pose is deceptively simple. Five minutes of Savasana removes mental and physical fatigue and soothes the sympathetic nervous system.

Note that while I am suggesting that you do this before bed, it can be done at any time. It does not require setting up; all you need is a folded blanket or pillow for your head. And it can be done anywhere.

Remember that knowing how to relax is a skill, something you learn. The props and other restorative poses I'll teach you are all refinements of this basic pose, helping you to have different experiences and sensations of being fully relaxed. This Savasana is where all yoga practitioners—even the most advanced practitioners—begin and return to again and again.

SAVASANA

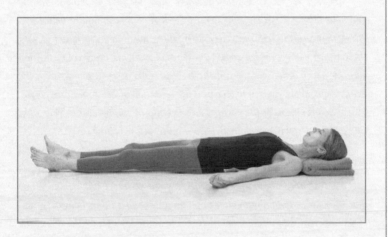

1. Lower the lights in the room.
2. Lie on the floor or on a yoga mat if you have one. Allow your feet to rest about 12 inches apart.
3. Support your head on a folded blanket or towel. As in the photograph, extend the back of your neck, bring your chin slightly down, and let your throat be soft. You want the head support to be easy, so that it is not straining your neck but emphasizing and supporting the natural curve and shape of your cervical spine. Let your feet and legs roll out into an easy, relaxed position. Extend your arms to the sides at an angle, knuckles down, palms up, hands relaxed.

(continued on next page)

As with all other yoga poses, make this pose yours, in your space and in your time. After you have set up, rest for a minute or two and then start to notice what you are feeling. Notice the sensation of the backs of the legs— your heels, calves, backs of the thighs, and buttocks—being completely supported. Allow your legs to sink even more into the floor. Be receptive to all of the sensations in your body. Notice how your back feels. Can you feel your shoulder blades and other parts of your back in contact with the floor? How do your head and neck feel? Let all the weight of your head be supported on the blanket.

Let your face relax, eyes closed. Make sure that your teeth are not biting and your tongue is not pressing against the roof of your mouth or your teeth. Allow your arms to rest completely, as if falling away from the center of your chest. When you get carried away by a series of thoughts, bring your attention back by noticing the sensation of the back of your body in contact with the floor. Again, allow yourself to give into the sensation of being fully supported. When you come out of the posture, do so gently by rolling over to your right side and comfortably resting there for a minute, before getting up.

If this is all you can do, it will be enough to get you started, and you will get results. Practice Savasana as often as possible for at least 10 minutes.

Special note about the restorative yoga poses: *I will be suggesting that you practice certain restorative poses on certain days throughout the course of this program. But please know that if either of today's poses—or any of the future poses I will be teaching you—feels good and you want to integrate them into your daily pulse, by all means go ahead! You cannot overdo them.*

Week 2

Move

*Life is movement. The more life there is, the more flexibility there is.
The more fluid you are, the more you are alive.*

—Arnaud Desjardins

When we take sugar and processed foods out and begin to ease the tension in our muscles, it revives us. But it also makes us more sensitive to how much physical discomfort and mental stress we have. After a week on the Spent restorative program, most people's bodies and minds have begun to wake up—but for many, what they wake up to are some pretty cranky bodies. The best way to soothe a sore, stiff body is to get it moving.

As you continue to not eat sugar, artificial sweeteners, and processed foods, this week we will look at the ways in which you move—posturewise and exercisewise—and modify the way you stand, sit, and work out by using proper alignment in a way that feeds you rather than fatigues you. We will also take gluten out of your diet, as gluten, a mixture of gliadin and glutenin proteins found in wheat, rye, and barley, can throw the digestive system out of balance, making our bodies feel tired. And we will add a multivitamin supplement that will give your body the nutrients it needs to adjust to its new rhythm.

By the end of these first two weeks, you will feel more as if your body is a warm, comfortable, and energized place in which to live.

DAILY BEAT 8

PRACTICE GOOD POSTURE

Many of my patients look at me with surprise when I tell them that maintaining good posture or alignment is essential to help them become less Spent. Just as you are now striving to achieve balance and rhythm with your food, you need to find it in your body. Here's why: when your structure is properly aligned, your body exerts less energy keeping itself straight, and you have more energy available to invest in daily activities.

When you're misaligned, your muscles become strained and exert stress on other internal organs. To preserve and increase your energy, you need to try to perfect your alignment as much as possible to end subtle muscle imbalances.

For example, if you work at a computer, you may find that as the day progresses your shoulders slump forward and your head moves closer to the screen. When this happens, your chest muscles shorten, your upper back becomes overstretched, and the deep neck flexors on the front of the neck contract as the head comes forward. Over time, these imbalances literally become your new compromised posture as your body adapts and compensates. The fascia (remember the fascia?) constricts, tightening all the soft tissues. Your muscles and tissues strain to work harder (in the upper back, for example) or not work (in the chest). Your spine is pulled out of line, and eventually your muscles become used to their misalignment. As a result, your structure is held in place by overextended muscles. The flow of blood is disrupted, and eventually, so is your muscles' ability to contract and relax properly.

Much of the musculoskeletal pain I see in my practice (and I see a lot because I practice acupuncture)—including rotator cuff injuries, headaches, and neck and back pain—is related to poor posture and the resultant constricted fascia. Rounded shoulders, a rounded upper back, a tight, restricted chest, and a forward head position create a huge strain on the neck.

These positions also restrict the normal movement of the shoulder. Even wrist and elbow pain can result from a postural imbalance.

If you feel tired or strained or get injured performing routine tasks, your ideal posture has probably been compromised. Over the next few weeks, I will be introducing a series of exercises to help you improve your posture. Some will help you with posture, some will help you release your strained muscles (the Ultimate Neck and Shoulder Release does this), and some will help you learn how to strengthen your core, which, when functioning properly, makes movement efficient and easy.

If you practice the suggested posture exercises and the release exercises with any kind of regularity, your body will gradually ease back into its ideal posture. Over time, practicing both kinds of exercises will reeducate the body so that it can move with more structural integrity throughout the day. Your joints will move more freely, you'll be able to breathe more deeply, and you'll decrease your risk of pain and injury. As a result, your energy will improve as you start using more of the correct muscles to keep you upright because there will be more efficient use of your muscular system, with certain muscles not having to overwork and previously constricted ones working again.

To identify and target the muscles that need releasing and strengthening, do a Posture Check on the Floor. Here's how:

POSTURE CHECK ON THE FLOOR

Lie down on the floor. Your body should essentially assume the shape of the basic Savasana (page 75) without a blanket under your head. Spread your legs out so that they are at least hip distance apart. Then clasp your hands behind your neck, gently lift your head off the floor, and return it to the floor so that the neck is elongated and the chin is tipping very slightly toward your chest. Then allow your arms to rest on the floor so that your armpits feel open. Allow your palms to face up. Relax your belly. Close your eyes and take ten deep breaths. Inhale down to the toes and exhale up and out through the tops of your shoulders—just picture it.

(continued on next page)

Allow your body to feel completely supported by the floor.

Next, begin to scan your entire body—feet to head. First, notice what is touching the floor and what is not. The heels, the calves, the thighs, the butt, the middle of your back, the shoulders, the backs of the arms and hands, the back of the head. Take ten more deep breaths, inhaling and exhaling, allowing your body to relax and feel more supported. Mentally scan your body, noticing the small discrepancies between your left and right side. Maybe one foot is flopped out more. Maybe one knee feels tighter. Maybe one hip is more rotated—this imbalance usually travels down to the opposite foot and up to the opposite shoulder. Why opposites? The body is constantly trying to achieve balance. Maybe one shoulder is completely on the floor and the other is floating a couple of inches above it. Take your time and allow yourself to travel around, getting to know the cranky wrist or the fact that your chin tends to move toward your right shoulder.

Now, with awareness and precision, bend your knees and place your feet hip distance apart and flat on the floor so that your entire back is resting and supported by the floor. Take ten more deep breaths, inhaling down your body, exhaling up and out. Allow your rib cage to settle and your stomach to be soft. Allow your lower back to become broad. Once you have settled into this position, scan the back again, noticing if you find any new imbalances. Maybe the right side feels shorter than the left. Maybe one hip or knee feels easier when bent. Take your time.

When you are done, raise your right arm up by your ear and roll onto your right side, pausing there with your head cradled in your right arm. Take a few more breaths, and then bring yourself up to sit.

Before you head out for the day, take a moment and write down what you found. As you move about your day today, notice the way you sit, stand, and walk. Do you lean to one side? Do you put more weight on one foot? Do you swing one arm more? These observations are just more information for you to use and bring to the postural practices I'll be teaching you.

The Pulse

○ ● ● ○ ● ● ○ ● ● ○

○ Have another protein- and nutrient-rich breakfast. **Try the smoothie of the week, the Greena-Colada Avocado Smoothie on page 270.**

○ Don't forget to make lunch your biggest meal of the day.

○ Continue taking three to four breathing breaks throughout your day.

SLEEP BEAT

○ Do the Ultimate Neck and Shoulder Release on page 57.

● **Try the Spinal Reset.**

This morning you did a little postural research. Tonight we're going follow that up with a Spinal Reset, which I think is one of the most effective ways to get the body back into alignment. Aligning the spine before sleep allows your body to absorb and adjust to a better posture with ease.

SPINAL RESET

Find a space in your home where you can lie down and extend your arms out into a T shape. Take your foam roller (which, I hope, you bought last week), and lie down lengthwise on top of it, ensuring that both your head and hips are on the roller. To support yourself, place your feet on the floor hip width apart or wider, toes forward, feet parallel. Allow your arms to be relaxed and drape open with the backs of your hands resting easily on the floor, assisting

(continued on next page)

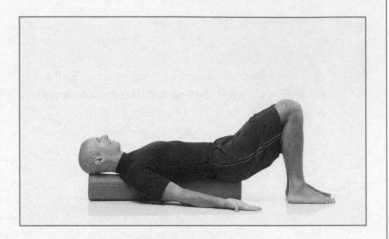

you with your balance. If your neck feels uncomfortable, place a small rolled towel under the back of your head.

Once you are settled and feel that your feet are planted, your arms are easy, and your entire spine is supported by the foam roller—from the back of the head to the tip of the tailbone—feel that the center of your body (your spine) is on an imaginary center line on the roller. Now surrender the weight of your body to the roller, inviting your breath to move deeply into the front, sides, and back of your torso, feeling the back of your rib cage expand into the roller.

Practice mindful breathing as you relax in this position for 3 to 5 minutes.

Then slowly roll to your right side, push the roller away, and roll back onto your back, relaxing in Savasana. Do another Posture Check on the Floor and feel how your spinal position has changed.

Benefits: Releases and resets tight glutes (butt muscles) and the erector spinae muscles, the muscles on either side of the spine. Relieves lower back pain, opens tight chest and shoulder muscles, and engages the core muscles (which we will be talking about later).

Caution: If you have a sense of vertigo—you feel as if you are falling backward or have a hot flash—carefully move out of the pose and rest on your right side until your equilibrium returns.

DAILY BEAT 9

TAKE GLUTEN OUT

As I discussed in the chapter "Prepare," restorative eating is about removing the foods that irritate and exhaust the system to let the body rest. Along with sugar and processed foods, I believe for many people, there is no greater drain on energy than gluten.

As I said in this week's introduction, gluten is a mixture of gliadin and glutenin proteins found in wheat, rye, and barley. Many people respond differently to grains with gluten in them than they do to other grains. Gluten can cause celiac disease, which is perhaps the most dramatic response. But it also seems to cause, in an ever-increasing number of people, an immune reaction, which can lead to a slow wearing down of one's system and feeling Spent. The folks who have this kind of gluten sensitivity suffer chronically from a vague unwellness, which doctors can't diagnose and/or don't know how to respond to.

According to Dr. James Braly and Ron Hoggan, M.A., in their book *Dangerous Grains*, it has been found that gliadin causes our immune system to react as though it is responding to a foreign body rather than a nourishing food.[1] It is believed that some people can produce a liver enzyme that helps break down this gliadin protein and then metabolize it. But many of us do not produce this enzyme, so the protein cannot be digested.[2] Instead, the gluten (think bread, pasta, etc.) is not broken down into smaller particles, and this bigger molecule or undigested protein then leaks through the gut wall and hits the bloodstream, where the immune system reacts and attacks it as though it were a foreign substance. Over time, fighting gluten makes our immune system tired and stressed, even Spent. Unfortunately, these potentially unhealthy grains are so cheap—and foods like bread and pasta are are so convenient—that they are the staple of most people's diets.

My experience over many years has shown me that eliminating gluten grains for a few weeks helps almost everyone who comes in to see me. If the body is expending less energy to deal with this hard-to-digest protein, it has more energy for other processes. Moreover, the liver and the digestive and immune systems are given time to rest and recover, which is why taking gluten out is part of my restorative process for healing Spent.

For the next five weeks, I will be asking you *not to eat* the following foods with gluten in them:

- *Grains such as wheat, barley, rye, bulgur, couscous, farina, kamut, kasha, semolina, spelt, triticale, and oats, and their derivatives, such as malt*
- *All flours containing wheat, oats, rye, malt, barley, or graham flour; all-purpose flour, white flour, wheat flour, bran, cracker meal, durum flour, and wheat germ*
- *Unless they specifically say "gluten free," breads, buns, rolls, biscuits, muffins, crackers, cereals containing wheat, wheat germ, oats, barley, rye, bran, graham flour, malt, kasha, bulgur, spelt, Melba toast, matzo, bread crumbs, pastry, pizza dough, pasta, rusks, dumplings, zwieback, pretzels, prepared mixes for waffles and pancakes, cakes, cookies, doughnuts, ice cream cones, pies, prepared cake and cookie mixes, bread pudding, bread stuffing or filling, anything that is breaded.*
- *Gravy and cream sauces thickened with flour, soy sauce, hydrolyzed vegetable protein, brewer's yeast (unless prepared with a sugar molasses base), yeast extract (contains barley), malted drinks, beer, ale, gin, whiskey, and drinks like Postum, Ovaltine, and Cocoamalt.*

Depending on your current diet, taking gluten out may be relatively easy or you may feel as if there is no food left on the planet. Fortunately, this feeling should last only a day or two, until you find things to replace your habitual grains. For instance, brown rice pasta is a great alternative to regular pasta, and, when toasted, Ezekiel sprouted bread is wonderful for sandwiches. The recipe section offers you many options—alternative foods, approaches to eating—to help you make the shift away from gluten. For most of us, leaving wheat (the gluten grain we eat the most) and all of its comforts behind takes a few days. Alternatives that you can eat include:

Amaranth	Montina
Arrowroot	Nut flours
Basmati rice	Organic corn in small amounts
Brown rice	Potatoes in small amounts
Brown rice pasta	Quinoa
Buckwheat	Sorghum
Ezekiel bread	Tapioca
Millet	Tef

Although Ezekiel bread is a grain bread, it is flourless and sprouted and, for most people, well tolerated. The problems people have with gluten are with the gluten lectins (found mainly in the seed coatings), which are destroyed in the sprouting process. Ezekiel bread is usually found in the frozen section of your natural foods supermarket.

A NOTE ON OATS

Historically, oats were not allowed on a gluten-free diet as they are a gluten grain.[3] However, new studies reveal that consumption of pure, uncontaminated oats does not cause a problem.[4] Unfortunately, most commercial oat products on the market have been cross-contaminated with wheat, barley, and/or rye, which occurs during harvesting, transportation, storage, milling, processing, and packaging. The good news is that there are specialty companies in North America and Europe that now produce pure, uncontaminated oat products. See page 311 for places to buy pure oats.

The Pulse
○ ● ● ○ ● ● ○ ● ● ○

- **Try cutting your gluten consumption in half today.** This means that if you have been eating toast with your breakfast, a sandwich for lunch, and some gluten-laden carb like pasta for dinner, you could have something like Ezekiel bread or preferably just your smoothie for breakfast, a protein-rich salad without a piece of bread for lunch, and a meal that includes another grain with your dinner—maybe grilled fish, brown rice, and steamed greens.

○ Continue taking breathing breaks to help cope with your cravings for bread and pasta.

● **Have a snack if you are having a midmorning sugar low or feeling sleepy in the afternoon. See Snack Attack, page 301.**

● **Continue refining your rhythm of eating by making a gluten-free meal for yourself tonight.** There are dozens of gluten-free meals listed in the back of the book and more at www.spentmd.com. Try cooking with quinoa or another grain you've never cooked before.

SLEEP BEAT

○ Turn off your TV, cell phones, and computers by 10 p.m.
● **Darken your bedroom.**

As I've said, back in the days of our ancestors, we rose with the dawn and slept when it became dark, and this cycle imprinted itself in our genes. But today, when it comes to light, we're overfed and undernourished—just as we are with food. During the day, most of us get artificial light from fluorescent bulbs instead of sunlight, so most of us miss out on getting the sun's vital vitamin D. And at night, when we need the dark to trigger melatonin production, we stay up too late and the excessive artificial light disrupts our body rhythms even more. So we have too much light when we don't need it (at night) and too little natural light when we do (during the day).

At night, if there is even the tiniest bit of light in the room, it can disrupt your circadian rhythm and your pineal gland's production of melatonin and serotonin. Cover or move your clock, use dark shades or drapes on windows if they are exposed to light, or wear an eye mask. There should also be as little light in the bathroom as possible if you get up in the middle of the night. Try keeping the light off when you go to the bathroom at night. Use a flashlight or night light. Believe it or not, as soon as you turn on a bright light, you immediately cease all production of melatonin for that night.

DAILY BEAT 10

VITALIZE YOUR DIET

Our mothers and fathers told us to eat our fruits and vegetables. When we asked why, they would say something like "Because they're good for you." Now you might even tell your own children to eat their fruits and vegetables. But most of us don't really know why fruits and vegetables—in a wide range of colors—are so essential to our health and well-being. Other than fiber, one of the key reasons our bodies need fruits and vegetables is that they are loaded with phytonutrients, which I mentioned briefly when I made the suggestion to add greens to your smoothie. Now I want to talk about them more.

Phytonutrients are biologically active substances that are responsible for giving plants their smell, flavor, and color. According to Dr. David Heber, the director of UCLA's Center for Human Nutrition, in his book *What Color Is Your Diet?*, phytonutrients also give plants a kind of immune system, protecting them from viruses, bacteria, harmful bugs, and too much sunlight. Scientists like Dr. Heber now believe that these same phytonutrients also protect the human body from disease by working as anti-inflammatory, detoxifying, hormone-balancing agents for the body.[5] The colors in our fruits and vegetables house more than twenty thousand beneficial chemicals.

These phytonutrients not only are full of antioxidants and other essential nutrients for your health but are essential for restoring rhythm because they offer a steady stream of messages about the environment. When animals eat plants in the wild, they get information about the change of seasons from them. This information is communicated to their reproductive systems and lets them know when to conceive so that their offspring have the best chance of survival. We are also part of nature, and we also get messages from our food, telling us about the natural world around us. The further removed foods are from nature, the fewer messages (if any) we receive.

So, in addition to what you eat, when you eat, and the size of the particular meal, eating fresh seasonal—and local, if possible—fruits and vegetables that are loaded with phytonutrients is an important way to eat to get back into rhythm. People suffering from Spent need as many of the healing properties that these colors bring as possible. The prescription for eating when Spent is to have a rainbow of color on your plate at every meal, beginning with a greens powder mix in your breakfast shake. This variety nourishes and heals us from the cells on up.

This said, no matter how many fruits and vegetables you eat, when you are Spent, it is highly likely that you will need to fortify your diet with supplements.

Many people believe, as do their doctors, that if they eat well they will get all the nutrients they need in their diet. But getting sufficient nutrients from your diet to beat Spent is not easy. Despite our belief that Americans have the best food supply in the world, most people don't obtain sufficient amounts of essential nutrients because our food is now grown in mineral-deficient soil. Further nutrient losses have been documented during the transportation, storage, and processing of produce all the the way from the farm to you.

Several years ago, U.S. Department of Agriculture researchers found that conventional nitrogen fertilizer reduced vitamin C levels in some food crops by as much as one third. So even if your intentions are good, it's often hard to walk out of a supermarket with truly nutritious fruits and vegetables. If the food you eat is mostly organic, you are better off, as a couple of smaller studies have reported that organic produce contains higher levels of vitamins and minerals than do regular supermarket foods.

Supplementation with concentrated food—like the greens powdered drink you are using—is the best way to ensure that you are getting optimal supplies of phytonutrients. But when you are Spent and living in an unnaturally polluted and stressful world, your need for other nutrients is also higher. After the greens powder, the first supplement that I suggest is a multivitamin. Yes, everyone should take a multivitamin because, as you have just learned, you can't get all the nutrients your body needs from the foods you eat anymore. And the simple act of taking a multivitamin every day can facilitate healing. There is no question in my mind that supplements can compensate for some of the damage that we do to ourselves and the lack of vital nutrients in the often devitalized food we eat today. I recommend them as long as you don't use the supplements to justify a poor choice of foods.

If you are skeptical about supplements and believe in the RDI—the Institute of Medicine of the USA's National Academy of Medicine's Recommended Daily Intake—you should know that most physicians (those who practice nutrition) and researchers consider the RDI an overly conservative and antiquated dietary standard. Separate studies of zinc and vitamins E, C, and D have all determined this.[6,7,8,9] The RDI was designed by the federal government as a guideline for "practically all healthy persons,"[10] but it's easy to question whether Americans can be considered healthy—and if you are Spent, you are definitely not "healthy."

In fact, in my opinion, the very concept of an RDI is flawed. Forty years ago, Roger Williams, Ph.D., who discovered the B vitamin pantothenic acid, developed the concept of "biochemical individuality." Williams contended that everyone needs the same nutrients but that we are highly individualistic in the amounts we need. For one person, 100 milligrams daily of vitamin C might be sufficient for health; for another, 3,000 milligrams. In other words, we are all so biochemically unique that our nutrient needs differ. These differences might even be as much as tenfold between people. I agree with Williams and Nobel Laureate Linus Pauling, Ph.D., who emphasized the concept of optimal nutrition, that we should provide each individual's body's cells with levels of vitamins and minerals that help them function at their best, rather than having a blanket menu of values for everyone.

Determining your optimal intake requires a little experimentation, but I have found that supporting the body with a few key supplements has helped my patients heal from Spent in leaps and bounds.

Remember, supplements won't make up for a bad diet. As the term suggests, supplements are supplements to—not replacements for—food. Always eat a good diet with loads of colorful, phytonutrient-rich fruits and vegetables, healthy fats, and good-quality protein. Use supplements to supplement the nutrients you just can't seem to get in your diet.

The Pulse

○ • • ○ • • ○ • • ○

- To ease stiffness and tension and wake the body up in the morning, practice the Wall Stretch (page 72) before work and maybe once in the afternoon while at work.
- Take a multivitamin. *Note:* Supplements are not regulated, so individual manufacturers are responsible for standards of safety and correct labeling (what is stated on the label should be what's in the product). I use only brands that I trust and have experience with. These products are made from high-quality ingredients and have proven safety and efficacy. All the products I recommend meet these high standards and are produced in an FDA-registered drug-manufacturing facility. See www.spentmd.com for resources.
- Have a lunch loaded with color—a substantial salad or a stir-fry with lean protein.
○ Continue to follow the Spent restorative eating program, liberating your body from sugar, artificial sweeteners, processed foods, and gluten.
○ Maybe try the Ultimate Neck and Shoulder Release (p. 57).

SLEEP BEAT

○ Darken your bedroom completely or use an eye mask.
- Before bed, try the Ultimate Foot Massage. Let's face it: our feet are abused. Beyond all the walking and running that we do throughout the day, many of us force our feet into uncomfortable or unsupportive shoes. Our feet (and entire bodies) suffer as a result. This is not good. For quick relief and repair, try this foot massage with tennis balls. It's almost as good as a pair of well-trained hands!

ULTIMATE FOOT MASSAGE

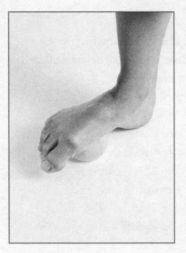 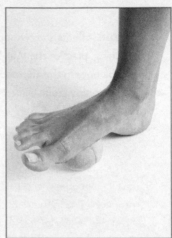

1. *Stand on your mat or carpeted surface with a tennis ball under the ball of one foot.*

2. *Gently press your body weight into the tennis ball. Slowly open and close your foot over the tennis ball, flaring your toes when you open them and squeezing like a fist when you close.*

3. *Repeat 5 times in one area, then move to a different part of the foot. Stop on any area that is tender, apply as much pressure as you can bear, and hold it for a few seconds.*

4. *Move on to the next area of tenderness and hold it. Continue until you have "rolled" every area of the foot.*

5. *When you are finished with one foot, stand with both feet on the floor and feel the difference between the two feet; it's pretty remarkable. Then do the other foot. Interestingly, when your feet feel relaxed, your whole body will too.*

Benefits: *Releases tight muscles and fascia in the feet, reduces strain and pressure on toes and toe joints from wearing shoes, and improves balance.*

Caution: *It will be painful in certain spots. That is normal, but if you feel any sharp pain, stop.*

DAILY BEAT 11

BIRDWINGS

"Birdwings" by Rumi

Translated by Coleman Barks with John Moyne

Your grief for what you've lost lifts a mirror
up to where you're bravely working.

Expecting the worst, you look, and instead,
here's the joyful face you've been wanting to see.

Your hand opens and closes and opens and closes.
If it were always a fist or always stretched open,
You would be paralyzed.

Your deepest presence is in every small contracting
                                        And expanding,
The two as beautifully balanced and coordinated as birdwings.

This process of adding and subtracting and subtracting and adding can be challenging, uncomfortable, even scary—especially if snack foods, sugar, and bread were what you used to comfort you in times of stress. But it is important to remember—again and again—that the stress of not eating them is not nearly as stressful as blasting your body with chemicals that you are not genetically designed to metabolize. By taking sugar, processed foods, hydrogenated fats, and gluten out of your diet, you are easing your body's total stress load. And by finding your eating rhythm—particularly having protein and good fats for breakfast and making lunch your biggest meal, adding more color to your diet, using your breath to ground you, and practicing restorative yoga and other release techniques, you are giving your body what it needs to begin to regenerate. Then you can find your essential pulse of expansion and contraction that Rumi is talking about so that you will take flight.

The Pulse

○ • • ○ • • ○ • • ○

- Check in with your rhythm of eating. Are you getting enough protein and healthy fats in the morning? Is lunch your biggest meal of the day? If you normally eat lunch or dinner out or take out from a restaurant, make sure that you are getting everything you need—protein and vegetables (especially dark greens like arugula, kale, spinach, and broccoli)—so that your body is truly well fed. Are you having a healthy snack when your energy drops in the late morning or afternoon?
- ○ Begin taking a multivitamin with your morning smoothie.
- ○ Do Spinal Reset (page 81) before heading off to work.

SLEEP BEAT

- Try Chair-Supported Savasana for ten minutes.

CHAIR-SUPPORTED SAVASANA

For whatever reason, just looking at this picture makes me sigh and relax. I suspect it is because my legs and lower back know how good this feels—instant physical relief and release. There really isn't a better pose for someone with back pain. The support of the chair gently nudges the lower back to open up, broaden, and release. Simultaneously, the hips and groin release and soften the belly. What can I say? It is so easy to do and another great way to prepare for sleep.

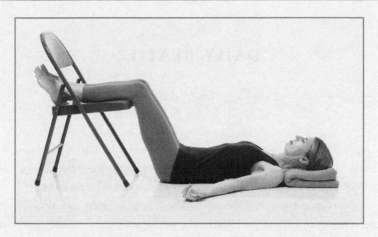

Look at the photograph and notice how the head is supported in the same way it was in the basic Savasana. It is important not to let the chin tilt up and the back of the neck shorten. Rather, the back of the neck extends and lengthens and, as a result, the chin comes down a little, so that the face is tilted downward slightly, as in the photograph. The face, eyes, and shoulders are easy and soft.

If you don't have a chair with a hole in the back like the one in the picture, use a regular chair turned sideways. Notice the angle of the thighs. Adjust your legs so that you have the sensation of their being fully supported and "falling" away from you onto the chair. This will give the groin and lower back (lumbar spine) a great sense of relaxation. Rest and breathe in this position for at least 10 minutes. To come out of the pose, place your feet on the edge of the chair, pause, then bend your knees in, roll over to the right side, and rest there for a full minute before getting up. Allow your head to be heavy, coming up last.

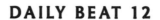

DAILY BEAT 12

START TAPERING OFF
CAFFEINE AND ALCOHOL

I know, I said that it was all downhill after the sugar, which for most people is the hardest. But stopping caffeine—particularly coffee—can also be excruciating. Fortunately, if you follow my plan, it doesn't have to be.

Every year there is some report about why caffeine and alcohol are good things to have in our diet. In the next breath there is another report countering the argument, saying that coffee and alcohol are essentially evil and incredibly unhealthy. Let me explain why I think you should avoid caffeine and alcohol if you are Spent.

Caffeine is a powerful stimulant with a half-life of typically seven hours. That means that seven hours after you drink it, half of it is still in your body. But for some people the half-life may be much longer, especially if they take a medication like an oral contraceptive, have liver problems, or are getting older. Caffeine, even in small doses, blocks sleep neurotransmitters. If you have a problem with sleep, I suggest you cut out coffee and any caffeinated beverages completely (even in the morning). Moreover, caffeine is a problem because it excites the adrenal glands, which help regulate your body's stress levels and are already overused from our overstimulated, hyperstressed lifestyles. It also throws off your body's circadian rhythms, and this effect seems independent of its effect as a stimulant. Remember, caffeine is not just in coffee. It's in sodas and other soft drinks, tea, even some herbal teas, chocolate, and some medications (Anacin and Excedrin, for example). There's a little caffeine even in decaffeinated coffee.

Alcohol is equally disruptive to our body's sleep rhythms. It is important to note that while alcohol initially has a sleep-inducing effect, when it is broken down by the body, it can lighten sleep and causes frequent and early awakening. Alcohol interacts with gamma-aminobutyric acid

(GABA) receptors, blocking the brain's oxygen sensors. This process cuts oxygen intake and complicates sleep conditions relating to sleep apnea. Alcohol is also high in sugar, which, as you know, is detrimental to those who are Spent.

If the notion of starting your day without coffee or ending it without a glass of wine seems unthinkable, I have a plan that should help even the most addicted caffeine addicts slowly taper their intake and those who like to drink ease off alcohol.

Here's how it goes:

Caffeine:

Day one: Today, have your normal amount of coffee. We have already axed soda from your diet because of its sugar. But if you're still thinking that diet soda is okay, it is not—because of the harmful artificial sweeteners and the caffeine. Quit soda now.

Days two to five: Blend your coffee 50–50 with decaf. Drink that for four days.

Day six: Have 25 percent regular coffee, 75 percent decaf for one day.

Day seven: Start drinking pure decaf.

Alcohol:

Day one: Today, have your normal amount of alcohol.

Days two to five: Cut your alcohol consumption in half. Drink this way for four days.

Day six: Stop drinking for three weeks.

Both these plans should reduce your physical cravings and ease your withdrawal. Drink plenty of mineral water to help flush your system. You can also enjoy two or three cups of green or black tea every day. These contain a very small amount of caffeine, which may take the edge off your symptoms.

As we go along, I will remind you of what you should be drinking. For now, enjoy your last fully caffeinated, alcoholic day.

The Pulse

○ ● ● ○ ● ● ○ ● ● ○

- **Commit to the idea that tomorrow you are going to begin tapering off coffee and alcohol.**
- ○ Try another smoothie recipe (see recipes starting on page 269).
- ○ If you are still having sugar cravings, continue taking 1,000 milligrams of glutamine every 4 to 6 hours.
- ○ Continue taking a multivitamin.
- **Remember to take your time while eating. Don't inhale your food, inhale your breath.**
- **Continue working on improving your posture and releasing physical tension; do the Wall Stretch (page 72) before work.**

SLEEP BEAT

- ○ To eliminate EMF radiation and brain stimulation, turn your TV, cell phones, and computers off by 10 p.m.
- ○ Make sure your bedroom is dark.
- **As I've said before, improving your sleep is the best way for people who are Spent to restore their health. One of the simplest (and most environmentally friendly) ways to improve sleep is to turn the thermostat down and keep your bedroom cool.**

Sleeping in a cooler bedroom supports our circadian rhythms. As we have discussed, from the beginning of time, people have awakened to morning light and fallen asleep in evening darkness. This is the normal cycle: energized during the day and sleepy at night. Part of the internal body clock's system is to change temperature.

Here's how it works: As the day progresses, our body temperature, which starts out low, begins to rise, as does our metabolism. As daylight wanes, our body clock cuts back on the active, energetic hormones, our body temperature begins to fall, our metabolism slows down, and we begin to wind down. As the light continues to fade, our body clock signals the pineal gland to convert serotonin into melatonin, and we become more lethargic. As melatonin and other sleep hormones increase, our temperature continues to drop, and we start thinking about withdrawing. It becomes difficult to stay awake or be active. This is the best time to fall asleep. And our body temperature continues to drop as melatonin is released into the bloodstream.

Sleeping in a cool room reflects our body's own natural rhythm of cooling for sleep. A sleeping temperature of 60° to 65° F. is best for most people, even in the dead of winter. In hot weather, use a floor or ceiling fan to create a breeze or an air-conditioner set at about 70° F., because this lower temperature encourages the production and release of sleep hormones.

DAILY BEAT 13

DO RESTORATIVE EXERCISE

In the introduction, I mentioned that I believe that our idea of exercise has become completely distorted. It sometimes feels as if there are only two modes: fanatical exercisers who work out once if not several times a day, pushing their bodies to extreme limits and exhausting themselves. Then there are those who are marathon sitters, who torture their fascia, knees, hips, shoulders, and neck with immobility. Being either too active or too sedentary is not healthy. My guess is that a lack of moderation in the field of exercise, no matter which camp you fall into, is part of what has led you to Spent.

If the idea of *moderate* exercise—whether you're a couch potato or a gym rat—makes you want to skip this beat, please don't. We're going to accomplish something with exercise in this book that's probably different from any approach you've ever tried before. The exercise regimen (for lack of a better word, because this program is far more flexible than the typical exercise regimen or any regimen, for that matter) in this book is going to help your body heal. For those of you who haven't moved in a while, yes, you *will* find the time, and no, it's not going to hurt. And for those of you who are terrified of letting go of your daily exercise regimens and think they are the only thing holding you together, think again. In many ways, your way of exercising could be one of the main reasons why you are Spent.

For example, Elizabeth, a driven stockbroker and workout fanatic, came to see me, at her wit's end and demanding a "quick fix." She told me she would get up at 5 a.m., pull on her exercise gear, and head to the park to run for an hour or more. On rainy or snowy days, she'd jog on her treadmill for ninety minutes. She complained that she didn't get her runner's high anymore. She couldn't understand why, because, in the past, exercise had been her feel-good, stress-relieving savior. These days she tired easily and had troubling muscle pains after exercising. Elizabeth didn't realize that the way she exercised was actually breaking down her system. I explained that exercise can be a stress on the body, especially if it is too intense. This kind of exercise stimulates the body's fight-or-flight response, which is there to help us respond to life-threatening situations. Essentially, your body reacts to Elizabeth's kind of exercise the way it would respond if you were in a car crash. It responds by pumping cortisol, which is a steroidlike substance it uses to give you the strength to survive a critical situation. As you might imagine, our bodies are not designed for continual overload, which is what Elizabeth and those who exercise like her are doing to their bodies when they exercise too rigorously. I've also had patients like Sandra, who are the complete opposite of Elizabeth. Sandra is a fifty-year-old art dealer who hated exercise and "had no time for it." Sandra was actually Spent because she did *not* exercise. She came in to see me complaining that she was so tired that she could barely keep up with the demands of her job. She worried about the fatigue, aches, and pains that were taking the joy out of her gallery-hopping and partygoing lifestyle.

I gave her some of the release exercises to ease the tension in her neck, shoulders, and hips, and I started her on my restorative exercise program. In addition, I encouraged her to move whenever possible—to walk instead of taking cabs, use the stairs instead of taking elevators. Slowly but surely, Sandra's body began to come back to life. She had fewer aches and pains, had more energy, lost weight, and began enjoying her exercise sessions.

Yes, the body needs to be used—Sandra had no exertion, which strengthens the body. But it also needs to rest—Elizabeth did not give her body an opportunity to rest, so that it was chronically exerting and exhausting itself. They both needed to get back to basics by using the body in appropriate amounts.

Hundreds of years ago, our ancestors used their bodies to hunt, build homes, and harvest food. I believe that exercise should echo the bursts of energy followed by periods of rest that were our ancestors' natural way of life and are programmed into our genes. Our ancestors didn't hop on a treadmill and stay there until they'd finished reading their *Wall Street Journals*. For them, exercise equaled survival. They sprinted hard and fast to catch their prey, or they sprinted hard and fast to avoid becoming prey; then they stopped. They didn't run for extended periods for no good reason. Their bodies simply weren't designed to do so, and neither are ours. What we are designed for is short activity bursts followed by rest. If you watch children play or animals run, that's what they do: start ... stop ... start ... stop. And if you look at most Eastern exercise traditions, such as yoga or the martial arts, recovery is built into the routine. Strenuous periods are always followed by relaxation periods. Exertion, rest, and recovery are the body's essential natural rhythm for movement in the same way that eating a larger lunch and smaller dinner reflects our innate digestive rhythm. Or the way sleeping in a dark room mirrors our genetically programmed rhythm for sleep.

My prescription for using physical activity to heal Spent is to practice restorative exercise. The regimen resembles interval training, in which short bursts of intense exertion are followed by rest and recovery. But my version is less aggressive. In standard interval training, the higher-intensity levels last from two to five minutes and are followed by lower-intensity periods of an equal time. I believe this is a bit too strenuous for those who are Spent and really need to train their bodies to recover. I advise my Spent patients to begin by performing high-intensity exercise for one minute, followed by three to four minutes of rest or low-intensity exercise. These bouts of higher and lower intensity are repeated several times to form a complete workout. For example, spend thirty minutes alternating between walking briskly for a minute and walking at a relatively relaxed pace for three minutes. As you feel better, you can increase your high-intensity levels from one minute to two minutes and decrease your rest periods from three to four minutes to two to three minutes, and so on.

This kind of exertion alternating with rest periods actually triggers the parasympathetic nervous system to activate the relaxation response, which is the opposite of the fight-or-flight response. Instead of stressing our bodies with movement, we are actually using movement to relax them! And the more we train our bodies to relax and recover from stress, the more they will begin to relax automatically, switching off the harmful chemical cascade triggered by stress.

Perhaps the best news—for both camps—is that restorative exercise burns more calories. By increasing the intensity for short bursts at a time, you'll increase your metabolism and burn more calories than if you worked at a steady pace.

How to Practice
Restorative Exercise

No matter what kind of shape you are in, I recommend beginning your restorative exercise with walking. If you have been overexercising, you need to slow down. And if you have not been exercising, walking is the appropriate way to speed up.

Walking is one of the most primal movement patterns. Because walking became essential to our survival as we evolved from our ape ancestors into our present upright form, our bodies have developed in such a way that walking is integral to our health. When we walk, we coordinate the movement of our arms, legs, and torso. Hundreds of calorie-burning muscles come into play—not only the muscles you'd expect, such as leg and arm muscles, but also internal muscles such as the psoas. The psoas is one of the body's major core muscles that is shortened by sitting (can cause knee and hip pain) and is lengthened and strengthened by the movement of walking. A daily walk burns calories, increases metabolic activity, helps counteract postural imbalances, and massages your internal organs. That's right, walking actually massages your internal organs. It also strengthens the abdominal walls and improves your breathing. Moreover, walking outside on uneven terrain is even better for you. It stimulates varied movement patterns, improving balance and coordination. Maybe there's a nature trail near your house with a choice of walking loops of varying distances. Of all the exercise available to you, I cannot think of a better cure for Spent than the combination of restorative yoga and restorative walking. If you're in good shape, you can incorporate short bursts of jogging into these brisk walks. Walk or jog briskly for a minute, then slow down for three.

All this said, though walking is the ideal mode of exercise for recovery from Spent, if you can't stand walking or it is physically impossible for you, you can do restorative exercise while swimming or using a recumbent bike or an elliptical trainer. For a more in-depth program and discussion of restorative exercise, go to www.spentmd.com.

Finally, let me offer you a few tips as you head out the door. This all may seem like common sense to you, but because it is common sense, I believe it is worth saying:

1. Consistency is essential for recovery. Whether you are an Elizabeth or a Sandra, not practicing restorative exercise on a regular basis won't serve either of your needs. Practicing restorative exercise needs to become a habit, something you can't live without, like sleep. Make the time and do it.

2. Don't exercise after 8 p.m. At a late hour, exercise will interfere with your ability to fall asleep. I believe that for many people, afternoon exercise helps restore rhythms best, but for most of us, it's more convenient to exercise in the morning. Since you're more likely to give up on a program if the timing is inconvenient, opt for morning exercise if it makes it easier to stick with your program.

3. Exercise is wonderful when it comes to relieving the stress, headaches, and overall detox process—particularly with caffeine.

4. Don't overdo it. We are trying to get you feeling un-Spent, not more Spent. It is important to remember that if you feel tired after moving or are so winded that you cannot talk, you have pushed your body too far. Don't stop or give up; just cut back a little and build up again more slowly.

The Pulse
○ ● ● ○ ● ● ○ ● ● ○

- Start your restorative exercise program. Remember: the key to a restorative exercise practice is short bursts of exertion followed by recovery. Start walking at a high intensity for 1 minute, followed by low intensity for 3 to 4 minutes. Do this for 30 minutes. If you can, do it outside. If slowing down and doing only 30 minutes of walking or swimming terrifies you, try this program for a week and see how you feel. I promise you that you will not lose strength, agility, or endurance. In fact, you will gain in all three areas! If 30 minutes seems like too much, it can be broken up into three parts. Three 10-minute segments of exercise are fine—park your car a bit farther from your destination, take the stairs, get off the subway or bus one stop away; even walking around the mall, doing housework, working in the garden, and so on can work.

- Today, blend your coffee 75 percent caffeinated and 25 percent decaffeinated.
- Keep yourself energized by having a piece of fruit, nuts, or trail mix (see page 301) midmorning and midafternoon.
- Drink half of your normal alcohol consumption today.
○ Continue to follow the Spent restorative eating program, liberating your body from sugar, artificial sweeteners, processed foods, and gluten.
○ Continue taking a multivitamin.

SLEEP BEAT

○ Keep your bedroom cool. Turn the thermostat down.
- Try this version of a Supported Savasana. This version uses blankets to lift and open the chest. It is particularly nurturing and soothing to the nervous system.

SUPPORTED SAVASANA

As in the photograph on the next page, you will need two yoga blankets folded to a size of at least 28 inches long and 9 inches wide. Place one on top of the other with a folded blanket or a pillow for your head. If you do not have Mexican yoga blankets, a sofa cushion or something similar will probably work as the support under the chest.

Start by sitting upright with the back of your buttocks up against the end of the blankets. If your back is sensitive, move 3 inches away (see the photograph). Lie back, being careful to be centered on the blankets. Extend the back

(continued on next page)

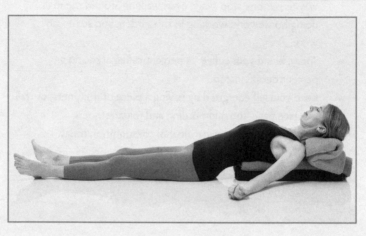

of your neck and adjust the blanket under your head so that it supports your neck as well. Take your time and set yourself up so that your body's position feels clear and your body feels completely at ease.

This pose relaxes the diaphragm and has a very healthy effect on the breathing as well as a soothing effect on the nervous system. It should feel different from the basic Savasana because it is lifting and supporting your chest. Again, allow yourself to take that support; let all your weight be supported by the floor and the blankets. If your breathing feels uneven or you are very anxious, occasionally take a slightly deeper breath and make a long, slow exhalation, at the same time feeling the back of your body and the supportive pressure of the blankets. When you begin to feel more relaxed, allow your eyes to fall shut and allow your breathing to be easy—not forced or controlled in any way. Rest and allow the pose to do the work.

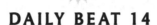

DAILY BEAT 14

DON'T SHOULD ON YOURSELF

I have a friend who says, "Don't should on yourself." I must confess that I need this advice as much as my patients do. In this day and age, it is very hard not to fill up our lives with shoulds. I should be working harder. I should be making more money. I should be spending more time with my children, boyfriend, family, friends. I should be exercising more. But this "shoulding" is a form of negative thinking. "Should" thought patterns load our brains, bodies, and lives with more to think about, more to do, and more emotions to handle, which ultimately adds more stress and makes us feel more Spent.

So today's assignment and reading are short and sweet: don't should on yourself today. The daily beats are getting longer, and, depending upon your tendency to underdo or overdo, you may be starting to feel bad about yourself because you haven't begun the restorative exercise (even though you know you should). Or you may be feeling bad about yourself because you missed one nighttime beat. No matter what, instead of shoulding on yourself, do something you love doing instead.

For the last two weeks, you have spent the bulk of your energy focusing on the physical body; however, your mental and emotional body needs relief too. The power of things that bring joy into our lives cannot be overstated. Laughter, companionship, or just doing something you adore has an incredible amount of healing power. I don't want to say too much because I want you to have as much time for yourself today as you can get.

The Pulse

○ • • ○ • • ○ • • ○

○   Try another breakfast smoothie.

●   **Drink 50 percent decaf with 50 percent caffeinated coffee.**

- Cope with the caffeine withdrawal by taking as many breathing breaks as you need to.
- Continue drinking half the amount of alcohol you'd normally consume.
- Do 30 minutes of restorative walking, alternating high-intensity walking for 1 minute with 3 to 4 minutes of recovery.
- Maybe go to the market and buy a bunch of Spent Superfoods that you've been wanting to incorporate into your diet.

SLEEP BEAT

- O Darken your bedroom completely or use an eye mask.
- Before you go to bed, practice the Spinal Reset (page 81) again. Then try the following twist. The rotation of the spine opens up the back and increases shoulder mobility.

SIDE-LYING SPINE ROTATION WITH ARM CIRCLES

Find some floor space in your house where you can stretch out.

Lie on your right side with your head, spine, and hips in one line. Bend your knees at 90 degrees so the knees are at hip level. Your arms should be at shoulder level on the floor in front of you.

Keeping your hips and knees still, slowly drag your top arm in a circle, starting down toward the hip, over the hip, on the floor behind the hips, gradually moving the arm overhead, then back to meet the other arm. Let the arm and hand rotate as they need to as you move the arm.

Repeat 5 times in one direction, then switch directions, moving the arm counterclockwise 5 times. Roll to your left side and move the right arm clockwise 5 times and then counterclockwise 5 times.

***Caution:** Those with lumbar disc herniations should avoid this exercise.*

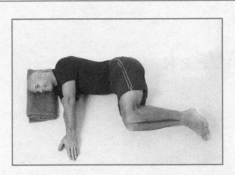

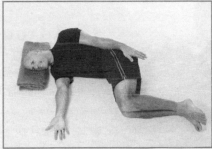

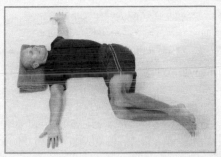

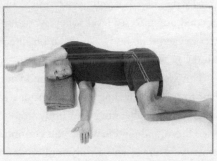

Week 3

Adapt

The state of our health reflects the food we eat, the exercise we take, the water we drink, the air we breathe and the quality of our housing and sanitation. I believe it also extends to our social needs and circumstances—the need to belong to a community, the need for meaningful work and daily purpose. The need in our lives for dignity and kindness, for self-respect, for hope and, above all, for harmony and, dare I say it, beauty. It encompasses the power of art, the healing properties of loving human relationships and the role of the human spirit. Human health is the sum of all these parts.

—Prince Charles

For years your body has toiled to adapt to a stressful, sleepless lifestyle. Now it is working to acclimate to a healthier way of living. Physiologically, it is a bit as if you were living at a high altitude and now you have migrated down to sea level, where your lungs and body are flooded with extra oxygen. The body can feel a bit discombobulated by this change in altitude.

This week is about giving you and your body more tools to help you adapt to this new feeling as you continue following the Spent restorative eating program, liberating your body from sugar, artificial sweeteners, processed foods, and gluten. While you continue to support your healing with restorative exercise and a daily multivitamin, I will also introduce you to adaptogens, herbs that help your body adapt to the body's imbalances, the perfect antidote to Spent. We will also explore things like getting more sun, spending time with friends, listening to music, doing more breathing work—all these help to support, ground, and bring us into connection with our surroundings and self. And we will take out dairy and unhealthy meats, which, at this stage in the process, are a bit like large encroaching weeds around a tree—they have a tendency to hinder rather than foster growth.

DAILY BEAT 15

ELIMINATE DAIRY PRODUCTS

Though cow's milk may be the perfect food for baby cows, it is not necessarily great for adult human beings. Although classic symptoms of dairy sensitivity and allergies are mucus production and respiratory and digestive symptoms—gas, bloating, and diarrhea or constipation—I also frequently see Spent patients who suffer from fatigue, joint pains, and other symptoms such as skin irritation, all of which go away when they stop dairy products.

The fact is that many people are sensitive or intolerant to cows' milk and many of them don't know it. The best-known and most common intolerance to cow's milk is lactose intolerance. Lactose intolerance affects up to 10 percent of adults and is associated with gas, bloating, and diarrhea after consuming cow's milk. Cow's milk contains a sugar called lactose that requires the enzyme lactase for its digestion. People with lactose intolerance are unable to digest lactose because they produce little or no lactase in their intestines. Undigested lactose then travels through the digestive tract to the colon, where it is fermented by the bacteria in the lower intestine, resulting in gas, pain, and bloating. Lactose intolerance does not involve the immune system and therefore is not considered a true food allergy.

Another less known but probably just as common reaction to cow's milk is from a protein called casein. People seem to have a hard time digesting casein. When casein is not properly digested, it gets into your blood and the immune system reacts accordingly. Interestingly, the casein in goat's and sheep's milk seems easier to digest for many of these same people. As I said earlier, although whey protein is derived from cow's milk, it is very unusual to have problems digesting it.

Even if we can metabolize cow's milk and have no sensitivity to it, the process of pasteurization takes out much of what is good for us in it. As you probably know, pasteurization is the process of heating milk to destroy potentially harmful organisms. Unfortunately, this process also eliminates many of the beneficial components of milk—immunoglobulins and the enzymes lipase and phosphatase. Pasteurization also takes out nearly 20 percent of the vitamin B6 in milk and kills *Lactobacillus acidophilus,* which is normally present in raw milk. These "friendly" bacteria that reside in our gut help us digest food and support our immune system, which, as you know, needs all the help it can get when you are Spent.

Then, to make matters even worse, we homogenize it. Homogenization creates fats that are foreign to most human digestive systems. There are serious questions about whether the human body can properly deal with these particular fats.

Though many people can tolerate dairy products, they are not necessarily the best thing for us—particularly in the large doses that most Americans consume. In terms of healing Spent, taking cow's milk out of your diet for a couple of weeks is a good idea because, no matter how your gut functions, not eating a food challenging to your digestive system allows the system to rest. Fortunately, there are still a few delicious cheese options: sheep's milk feta, goat cheese, buffalo mozzarella. Sheep's milk and goat's milk are much easier to digest and give us the same nutritional benefits, including calcium.

If you cannot live without cow's milk, I suggest you try raw cow's milk. This is illegal in many states, which claim that it is "dangerous" and "unsanitary." But my take on this is that these are the states with bigger interests and investments in and commitments to the pasteurization and homogenization processes. If you can buy raw milk products from a reliable local dairy farmer, I encourage you to try it. See the Weston Price Foundation Web site for more information: www.westonprice.org.

If you find products like Lactaid helpful, you probably are lactose-intolerant rather than sensitive to casein. Many lactose-intolerant people do find that they can tolerate yogurt because it is fermented and more easily digested and contains lactobacilli, which remove some of the lactose.

The Pulse

○ ● ● ○ ● ● ○ ● ● ○

- **Stop or seriously limit consuming cow's milk. This means most cheeses with the exception of sheep's milk feta, goat cheese, and buffalo mozzarella cheese. Rice milk and almond milk are both great alternatives to accompany your morning tea.**
- ○ Do 30 minutes of restorative exercise, alternating between high-intensity walking for 1 minute and 3 to 4 minutes of recovery.
- **Try the Smoothie of the Week, the Ginger Pear Smoothie on page 272.**
- **Continue drinking 50 percent decaf and 50 percent caffein-ated coffee today.**
- **Continue drinking half the amount of alcohol you normally consume.**

SLEEP BEAT

- ○ Turn off your TV, cell phones, and computers by 10 p.m.
- ○ Practice the Ultimate Foot Massage (see page 92).
- **Before you go to bed, practice Viparita Karani for ten minutes.** I have yet to meet someone who doesn't feel a sense of joy after ten minutes of this amazing restorative yoga pose.

VIPARITA KARANI (VI-PAR-EE-TAH CAR-AHN-EE): "INVERTED LAKE POSTURE" OR "LEGS UP THE WALL"

This is another refreshing restorative pose that you can do anywhere. It regulates blood pressure, refreshes the abdominal organs, and prevents varicose veins. It is great after air travel or a day on your feet. It is very easy to do.

First, grab a blanket and find a clear wall in your house. Next, lie on the floor so that your left hip is touching the wall. Bend your knees and then slowly roll down onto your side so that your right hip touching the wall and both hips and feet are touching the floor, as in the first photograph. Then bend

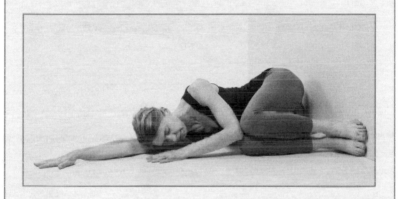

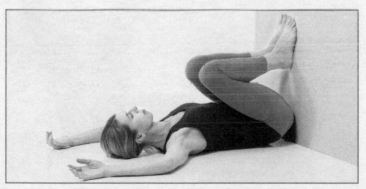

(continued on next page)

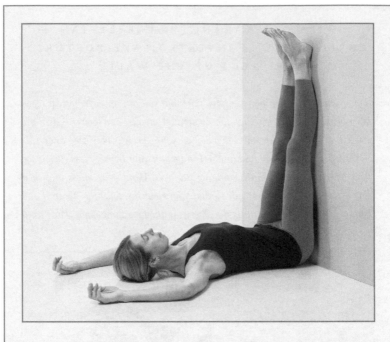

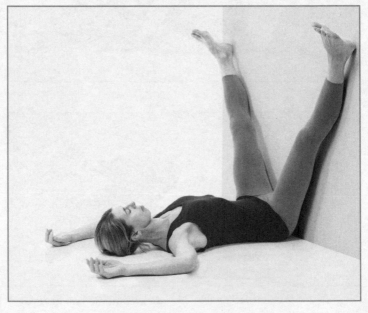

your knees into your chest, hug them in, and then swing around, bringing your legs up onto the wall. Your body should make an L, as in the third photograph. Your butt should be as close to the wall as your hamstrings will allow. If your head is on a hard surface, you may want to place the blanket under your head so that your chin is parallel with the floor. Move your arms out to your sides in a cactus shape. Keep your legs straight and, as with Savasana, relax your head, face, neck, shoulders, and belly. As a variation, while doing the pose, move your legs into a modest split for a minute or two, as in the fourth photograph. Stay that way for ten minutes.

Note: If you feel a slight tingling in your legs, this is normal. If it becomes painful, bring your legs down and take an easy cross-legged position with your legs still resting on the wall.

Caution: Do not practice this pose during menstruation.

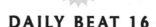

DAILY BEAT 16

DISCOVER THE POWER OF ADAPTOGENS

Botanical medicine has something to offer people with Spent that no expensive pharmaceutical can ever match. It's a group of herbs called adaptogens, which work a bit like a thermostat. When a thermostat senses that the room temperature is too high, it lowers it; when it senses that the temperature is too low, it raises it. Adaptogens can calm you down, yet boost your energy at the same time. Essentially, adaptogens help your body adapt to stress and resist fatigue. They work slowly over time and are safe to take long term. Western herbalists call these "tonic herbs," because taking them is like taking an old-fashioned tonic that makes you feel better all over. Though the effects may initially be subtle and take time to establish, they're real and undeniable—and are the perfect antidote to feeling Spent.

The word "adaptogen" was coined decades ago by the Russians during their extensive research on eleuthero (*Eleutherococcus senticosus,* formerly called Siberian ginseng). Back in the days of the Cold War, Russian scientists reportedly investigated eleuthero and other adaptogens to determine their ability to help the body deal with radiation poisoning. This work led to the knowledge that adaptogenic herbs help your body deal with the physical assault of stressful circumstances, enhance stamina and endurance, and strengthen immunity. The adaptogenic herbs I consider most important for helping defeat Spent include the following:

Asian ginseng (*Panax ginseng*) is one of the most valued (and expensive) medicinal plants in the world and has been for thousands of years. Ginseng is believed to affect the body by influencing metabolism within individual cells. It has been studied extensively for its ability to help the body withstand stress. Western herbalists say that it restores and strengthens the body's immune response, promotes longevity, and enhances the growth of normal cells. Research indicates that it promotes a sense of well-being, enhances performance (at higher-than-normal doses), and may protect against some kinds of cancer.

Dose: 100–200 *milligrams per day of a standardized extract (most standardized ginseng extracts supply approximately 4% to 7% ginsenosides). Or 1–2 grams per day of the dried, powdered root, usually taken in gelatin capsules.*

Caution: At the recommended dose, ginseng is generally safe. Occasionally it may cause agitation, palpitations, or insomnia. Consuming large amounts of caffeine with large amounts of ginseng may increase the risk of overstimulation and gastrointestinal upset. If you have high blood pressure, your blood pressure should be monitored when taking it. Ginseng is not recommended for pregnant or breast-feeding women.

Eleuthero (*Eleutherococcus senticosus*) is used in traditional Chinese medicine for muscle spasms, joint pain, insomnia, and fatigue. In Germany, its use is approved for chronic fatigue syndrome, impaired concentration, and convalescing after illness. Western herbalists note that it improves memory and feelings of well-being and can lift mild depression. It is great for people who work too hard and sleep too little.

Dose: 2–3 grams per day of the dried root.

Caution: As with Asian ginseng, eleuthero is generally safe. But occasionally it has been associated with agitation, palpitations, or insomnia in patients with cardiovascular disorders. If you have high blood pressure, your blood pressure should be monitored when taking it. Even though there is no evidence of harmful effects in the fetus from limited use by pregnant women, I generally don't recommend it for pregnant or breast-feeding women.

Ashwagandha (*Withania somnifera*) has been used for thousands of years in Ayurveda, the traditional medicine system of India. It has been nicknamed "Indian ginseng" because like Asian ginseng, China's king of herbs, it's used for helping increase vitality, energy, endurance, and stamina, promote longevity, and strengthen the immune system (although it is not related to ginseng botanically). Today herbalists often recommend it for people with high blood pressure, insomnia, chronic fatigue syndrome, and impotence associated with anxiety or exhaustion. It enhances endocrine function, especially the thyroid and adrenals. Ayurvedic healers have long prescribed the herb to treat exhaustion caused by both physical and mental strain. Most of my patients who are Spent and who take ashwagandha respond after a week or two by feeling warmer and having more energy. After a few weeks they often come back feeling stronger—and with an enhanced libido as a bonus.

Dose: 3–6 grams per day of the dried root.

Caution: Avoid during pregnancy and don't take if you are taking sedatives or if you have severe gastric irritation or ulcers. Also, people who are sensitive to the nightshade group of plants should be careful.

Rhodiola rosea acts like a hormone thermostat, especially as it pertains to cortisol, which, as you learned when we talked about sugar, is one of our main stress hormones. I believe the circadian rhythm of cortisol is usually, if not always, impaired when you're Spent. This means the cortisol level is either too high when it should be low or not high enough when you need more.

Getting your cortisol back into rhythm when you are Spent is crucial, and rhodiola helps balance the cortisol level in your body, raising or lowering it as needed. That's why this herb is particularly useful for treating Spent. What's more, rhodiola has demonstrated a remarkable ability to support cellular energy metabolism. It positively affects brain function, depression, and heart health. In my experience, most people with Spent who take rhodiola start feeling better within a few weeks to a month.

Dose: 200–600 milligrams per day of a Rhodiola rosea *extract standardized to contain 2% to 3% rosavins and 0.8% to 1% salidroside. Or 2–3 grams per day of the nonstandardized root.*

Caution: Avoid if you have manic depression (are bipolar). Rhodiola is not recommended for pregnant or breast-feeding women. Although unusual, at high doses rhodiola may cause insomnia.

You can take all of these adaptogens individually. If you were to choose only one adaptogen, I would recommend rhodiola. However, I have found that they work best when they are used together. Adaptogenic formulas are extremely effective. Look for one that has at least three of the above four adaptogens in one formula, making sure it has some rhodiola in it.

Although I think adaptogens are the perfect antidote to Spent, they should be used intelligently. I recommend taking them for three months and then taking a break for three weeks. If you feel you need them again after the three-week break, repeat the cycle.

The Pulse
○ ● ● ○ ● ● ○ ● ● ○

- Buy or order an adaptogenic formula or pick one or two individual adaptogens that you feel might fulfill your needs. For more information about some of my favorite formulas, go to www.spentmd.com.
- Make plans to see or talk to a friend tomorrow night.
○ Continue to follow the Spent restorative eating program, liberating your body from sugar, artificial sweeteners, processed foods, gluten, and dairy products.
- Drink coffee that is only 25 percent caffeinated.
- Stop drinking alcohol.
○ Do 30 minutes of restorative exercise, alternating between 1 minute of high-intensity walking and 3 minutes at a slower pace.

SLEEP BEAT

○ Keep the thermostat low to support your sleep hormones.
- Begin regulating your sleep schedule.

Nothing helps your circadian rhythms more than getting up and going to sleep at the same times every day. A change in your daily habits such as a short night's sleep can disrupt your circadian rhythms. People who regulate their sleep schedules give their bodies the opportunity to establish a rhythm. For instance, for someone who goes to bed at eleven and gets up at six, the body knows that it is going to need melatonin at eleven and serotonin and cortisol at around six, whereas someone who changes sleeping and waking times has a body that constantly needs to recalibrate, which tires it out. In a sense, a lack of schedule puts the body into a perpetual state of mild jet lag.

DAILY BEAT 17

HANG OUT WITH FRIENDS

My friends tell me I have intimacy problems, but they don't know me,
so who cares what they think?

—Garry Shandling

As with exercise, many of the people I see who are Spent are usually extreme in their social habits—they either are virtually hermits or haven't spent a quiet night at home in months. As you can imagine, neither of these tendencies is necessarily great for us. But spending quality time with friends and/or family is. In fact, I believe it is the most powerful natural mental and emotional salve we have.

Though many of us spend our days (and nights) with people, we are not necessarily emotionally fed by this kind of just-existing-in-the-same-space human contact and interaction. As Garry Shandling's quote suggests, the people we sometimes refer to as friends—our colleagues and casual friends—don't necessarily know us. There isn't an exchange of real worries, heartfelt laughter, and emotional victories. So I want you to make sure that you are getting real connection time—with friends, family, and loved ones. Silly talks, heart-to-hearts, laughter, and hugs are all very good for your well-being.

The idea that spending time with others is healing is not just some woo-woo concept. A group of molecular biologists at the University of California recently determined that loneliness can actually harm a person's health. The research team took blood from study subjects and found that the people who described themselves as lonely were also the people with the weakest immune systems. This said, your immune system is not going to erode from one night (or even a week or two) away from friends.

I believe that spending time alone is equally important, especially for those who tend to be overly social, exhausting themselves by giving too much. We all need time to breathe, think, and not talk. But when I talk about quiet time alone, it does not mean sitting in front of a TV. Healing alone time includes doing things like listening to music, walking in a park or on the beach, or pursuing creative endeavors, from playing music and writing to cooking or drawing and painting.

Finding a rhythm for time alone and time with friends is as important as finding your natural rhythm for eating and exercising. While there is not necessarily a genetic clock for this rhythm, it is essential for all of us to know others and to be really known. Our best friends, more often than not, notice that we are out of rhythm before we even do: "You seem off today. Is there anything going on?" This kind of simple question helps us pull our heads out of the sand and move back into rhythm with our truer selves.

The Pulse
○ ● ● ○ ● ● ○ ● ● ○

○ Do the Wall Stretch (page 72) first thing as a way to wake up and open up your body.

● Think about whether or not you need some contact with a friend or if a quiet night would be better for you. Depending on what you need, make plans for tonight to snuggle up with your partner, have dinner with a friend, or spend a quiet healing night alone.

● Begin taking the adaptogenic formula.

○ Continue taking a multivitamin.

● Stop drinking coffee, and continue not drinking alcohol.

● Take a day off from your restorative exercise, even if you have more energy. Let the energy build by taking a rest today.

SLEEP BEAT

○ Darken your bedroom completely or use an eye mask.

○ Keep working on regulating your sleep schedule.

● Our necks and shoulders can always use more relief. Neck and shoulder tension can cause a multitude of problems, including headaches and trouble focusing. As you probably know, headaches and neck and shoulder pain can really interrupt your sleep, which leads to fatigue and Spent. To relax and relieve some of this tension before bed, practice the Side-Lying Spine Rotation with Arm Circles (see page 108) and then try the Neck and Shoulder Release Using a Foam Roller.

NECK AND SHOULDER RELEASE USING A FOAM ROLLER

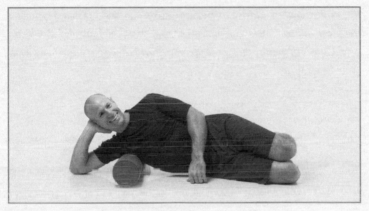

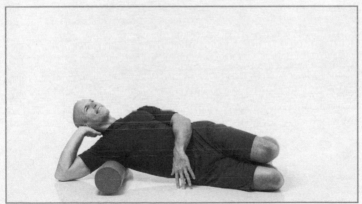

(continued on next page)

Rest the right side of your upper rib cage on the foam roller, just below the armpit, as in the photograph. Make sure that the outside edge of your shoulder blade is in line with the roller. Bend your knees and be sure that your head is supported by your right arm. Your left arm is on the floor in front of you for balance. Slowly tilt your body toward your front arm, then tilt it back toward the wall behind you. You should feel the roller contacting your shoulder blade and moving it side to side as you move. Pause on tender areas, hold for one minute, and then continue exploring other areas that need attention. When you have finished with your right side, release the left side.

__Benefits:__ Relieves round shoulders and neck strain from sitting at a desk. It also relieves pressure in the low back from sitting and increases mobility in the shoulder. This is an excellent exercise to assist in recovery from a frozen shoulder, a rotator cuff injury, low back strain, and rounded shoulders.

__Caution:__ Ensure that the foam roller stays below your armpit and away from breast tissue.

DAILY BEAT 18

LET THERE BE LIGHT

There is no greater healer of Spirit than the sun.

For the last twenty-five years or so we have been brainwashed by doctors, dermatologists, and skin care companies about the dangers of the sun. I do not agree with this hysteria. Just as we need darkness to support our sleep cycles, we need light—particularly morning sun—for our day cycles. The sun literally gets us going in the morning. We need its light to trigger our metabolism, alertness, and overall ability to function and perform.

Fortunately, in the last few years, the pendulum has swung back in this direction. Now it seems as if every month there is a new study documenting the beneficial effects of sunlight and vitamin D, which, as you know, we get from the sun. For instance, in one of these recent studies, researchers at the Moores Cancer Center at the University of California, San Diego (a very sunny place), concluded that almost 150,000 cases of cancer particularly colorectal and breast cancer—could be prevented each year by just ten to fifteen minutes a day of exposure to sunlight. Numerous other studies have supported this research, showing that modest unprotected exposure to sunlight helps the body produce the vitamin D it needs to keep bones healthy and protect against cancer, including skin cancer. Yes, you read that right.

Of course, repeated sunburns—especially in childhood and in very fair-skinned people—have been linked to melanoma. But there is no credible scientific evidence that *moderate* sun exposure causes skin cancer. I am not suggesting you slather on baby oil and lie in the sun for hours or go to a tanning salon, but getting some sun without getting a sunburn makes good health sense. Human beings evolved in and under the sun, and we are genetically engineered to get sun, not to live our lives indoors and pour on the sunscreen every time we do go outside.

Humans need the sun to regulate their circadian rhythms—stimulating their metabolism and daytime hormonal functions—and because they need vitamin D. Many health experts believe that 50 percent of Americans are deficient in Vitamin D.[1,2,3]

In fact, in one study, published in 2003 in the *Mayo Clinic Proceedings,* researchers in Minneapolis tested vitamin D levels in patients suffering from chronic nonspecific musculoskeletal pain, and 93 percent of them turned out to be deficient in vitamin D.[4]

Although it's called "vitamin" D, the substance is not really a vitamin. It is what is called a prehormone, as it is your body's only source of calcitrol (activated vitamin D). Calcitrol is the most potent steroid hormone in the body. Like all steroid hormones, vitamin D is involved in making hundreds of enzymes and proteins, which are crucial for preserving health and preventing disease. Vitamin D, which is a key nutrient for healthy bones, also serves as an anti-inflammatory, enhances muscle strength, helps insulin function, bolsters the immune system, and helps the body fight cancerous activity.

Because of its vast array of benefits, maintaining optimal levels of D is essential for your health. It's actually made in the skin after sun exposure, and unfortunately, without sun the body cannot manufacture its own. In fact, this is such an efficient system that most of us make 20,000 units of vitamin D after only twenty minutes of summer sun without suntan lotion. That's 100 times more than the government recommends per day! I believe that there must be a good reason why we make so much in so little time.

If you feel you aren't getting adequate amounts of sun exposure or are wary of the sun, you can take vitamin D supplements. If you would like to take a vitamin D supplement because it is just impossible for you to get outside and get twenty to thirty minutes of sun a day or you live in a place that is perpetually gray or cold, you should be tested by your doctor to see how much vitamin D you need. You can ask your doctor to order a test called 25(OH)vit D, also called 25-hydroxyvitamin D. You want your level to be at least 50ng/ml (or 120nmol/l) or higher. When buying supplements, make sure they are vitamin D3 and not vitamin D2, which is useless. If you do take vitamin D3 supplements, have your levels checked every three to six months, as too much can cause toxicity, though rarely. But please know that the best and safest way to get your daily dose of vitamin D is from the sun. Sun exposure doesn't cause vitamin D toxicity.

However, if you live in a cooler climate, supplementation during the winter months is probably necessary.

Vitamin D aside and no matter where you live and what it is like outside, it is important to get outside and get natural morning light to wake your body up and set your rhythm for the day.

The Pulse
○ ● ● ○ ● ● ○ ● ● ○

- Get thirty minutes of sun outside the peak hours—maybe while doing your 30 minutes of restorative exercise. Depending upon your levels of fitness and fatigue, you can increase the periods of intensity and decrease the periods of rest; for example, walking fast for 2 minutes and resting for 3.
○ To continue to nourish your body and help restore its balance, continue taking a multivitamin and an adaptogenic formula in the morning.
○ Continue to follow the Spent restorative eating program, liberating your body from sugar, artificial sweeteners, processed foods, gluten, dairy products, alcohol and caffeinated beverages.
- Buy full-spectrum lightbulbs for your house. Replace the bulbs in your house with full-spectrum lightbulbs now or as the old ones wear out. As I've said, most of us spend our days indoors with artificial or fluorescent lights. Even if there are many windows, the windows themselves block some of the 1,500 wavelengths present in sunshine from reaching our retinas and nourishing our brain and body. In most metropolitan areas, air pollution and haze are pervasive, blocking out the sunlight all year long. Many of us live in climates with winter weather that deprives us of essential sunlight. Fortunately, there is a simple solution: putting full-spectrum lights indoors helps you get benefits similar to those of sunshine. *Getting high-quality full-spectrum light indoors is essential if you are Spent and not getting adequate natural sunlight.* Not only will you sleep bet-

ter, but you will notice that your concentration, mental clarity, mood, and energy improve. And you won't get sick as often. Let the sun shine in!

Full-spectrum bulbs are widely available. You can find them at most good hardware stores, or go to www.gaiam.com.

SLEEP BEAT

○ Continue to regulate your sleep schedule.

● To prepare for bed, practice your favorite version of Savasana for ten minutes: basic Savasana (page 75), Chair-Supported Savasana (page 94), Supported Savasana (page 105), or Viparita Karani (page 115).

DAILY BEAT 19

START EATING ORGANIC, GRASS-FED, FREE-RANGE MEAT, POULTRY, AND EGGS

If you are vegetarian, feel well versed in the benefits of free-range eggs, and do not want to read about meat, that's fine. Fast-forward to the Daily Pulse and then the Sleep Beat and check in with your eating. Those of you who do eat meat, read on.

Today, most commercially available meats are factory farmed because it's fast, convenient, and more profitable. But factory farming is creating a host of problems, including, I believe, contributing to the epidemic of feeling Spent.

Originally all cattle were fed on grass and shrubs, which is what they were meant to eat. Grazing animals such as cows, sheep, goats, and bison possess a rumen, or second stomach, which is like a fermentation tank. In this rumen, bacteria convert grasses, shrubs, and other plants into protein and fats. When you feed these ruminants grains instead of grass, which is what happens at large factory farms, all sorts of problems occur. In particular, it makes their digestive tracts acidic and they develop subacute acidosis, which means the cows suffer from diarrhea and excessive salivation. This leads to such discomfort that the cows will do things like kick at their bellies, eat dirt, and stop eating to try to stop the diarrhea and salivation. We also know that this acidic environment in their stomachs encourages the development of *E. coli* bacteria. This is the reason why factory-farmed animals are given antibiotics—to compensate for this as well as their unsanitary and crowded living conditions.

Unfortunately, in treating for widespread subacute acidosis, farmers have learned that the antibiotics also help fatten the cows. In fact, according to the Union of Concerned Scientists (UCS), an estimated 70 percent of the antibiotics made in the United States are used to fatten livestock. I believe this is contributing to our Spent crisis. Public-health authorities have even linked low-level antibiotic use in conventionally raised livestock directly to greater numbers of drug-resistant infections in people—another ever-growing health crisis.

To make matters worse, switching ruminants from their natural diet of grasses to grains also lowers their nutritional value. Compared with grass-fed meat, feedlot meat contains more total fat, saturated fat, and calories. It also has less vitamin E, beta-carotene, and two health-promoting fats called omega-3 fatty acids and conjugated linoleic acid, or CLA.

This story of confinement, poor food, antibiotics, and lower nutritional value is also true for pigs, chickens, sheep, turkeys, and ducks. Unfortunately, even some organic products come from animals that are raised in confinement and fed grains. On the plus side, at least the feed for these "organic" meats and poultry doesn't contain restaurant waste, animal by-products, municipal garbage, bubble gum (yes, gum and garbage are commonly used), and poultry manure, as it does in regular feedlots. Nonetheless, beyond looking for phrases like "organic," "grass fed," and "free range," the best thing you can do is buy your meat, chicken, and eggs from a local farm or farmer whom you know. This is really the only guarantee that you are getting food that has been raised with care.

When you choose well-cared-for, local, organic grass-fed beef, lamb, bison, pork, or poultry, you're eating nutritious and healthy meats, as nature intended.

Great resources for more information are www.eatwild.com and www.themeatrix.com. Check them out.

The Pulse
○ • • ○ • • ○ • • ○

- Make a commitment to start buying local, grass-fed, free-range organic meat and poultry. This is for you, your family, and generations to follow.
- Do 30 minutes of restorative exercise, preferably outside, and at a pace that is simultaneously challenging but not exhausting.
- Continue taking an adaptogenic formula.
- Continue to not drink alcohol or caffeinated beverages.
- Make a meal using grass-fed, free-range organic poultry or

meat. Feel the difference. If your store or restaurant doesn't have it, ask if it can start carrying it. The more people ask, the more widely available it will be.

O   Remember not to should on yourself.

SLEEP BEAT

O   Continue to regulate your sleep schedule.

●   Before bed, pause and check in with how you are eating.

I keep asking you to refine your diet, taking more out and tweaking what you are eating—moving you more toward eating more and more local, organic whole foods. For most of us, this is an enormous shift.

My patients tell me that one of the toughest parts of integrating these changes is to find a new set of recipes and foods that are easy to make and tasty. As I've said before, my wife, Janice, and I have assembled ideas and recipes in the back of this book. But I also urge you to go to your local bookstore and peruse the cookbook section, looking for recipes and meals that speak to you. Maybe you want more Italian-influenced food or more Indian-influenced food. Finding the foods we like and can eat on a daily basis makes finding a rhythm for eating them much easier. So think about the meals you have been having and when you have been having them. Have you looked forward to them? Have they been satisfying? Do you like your snacks? Do they refuel you? How do you feel after eating a snack? What colors have you been eating? What colors do you need more of? Do a little minievaluation of the past two weeks, and see where you think you could improve and feed your palate and body more.

If you are a vegetarian, are you getting enough protein while you are on the Spent restorative eating program? Are you incorporating the sheep's milk feta, goat cheese, and buffalo mozzarella, eggs, nuts, beans and rice, and protein shakes into your daily eating rhythm so that you feel energized? Do you need to go to the market to stock up? Be sure that you are really nourishing your body.

DAILY BEAT 20

RETURN TO THE BREATH

Because meditation has such healing potential, I suggest that all of my patients find a meditation practice that suits them. As you probably know, practicing meditation does not mean sitting in a pretzel-like lotus position, chanting or worshiping some deity—it is not a religion—nor does it necessarily even mean sitting. I believe meditation can be anything you do with prolonged focused attention that helps you interrupt the usual ramble of worries, reflections, and projection in your head. You can walk and use your breath as your focus. You can cook and use the recipe as your focus. You can even knit, using the stitches as your focus.

Meditation is essentially restorative exercise for your mind. You *exert*—have a train of thoughts—*rest*—watch your breath, which then gives your brain a break from endless thinking. This process gives the mind a chance to *recover*. And when we go through this practice of thinking and then returning to the rhythm of our breath over the course of a few minutes, it triggers a kind of cascade effect throughout the body. Your muscles relax, more oxygen gets in, and tension moves out. As you can imagine, the more we can trigger the relaxation response, the less Spent we feel, which is why meditation is an invaluable tool for you.

But meditation doesn't just produce a positive physiological response; it also trains us to have a relaxed response to external stress. By training our minds to not always react to our thoughts, we learn to be less reactive to things like a person cutting us off on the road, your boss taking her stress out on you, or your child's tantrum. In my experience, after practicing meditation for some time, I have learned to take this type of experience less personally. If a person is rude on the train or someone is brisk with me on the phone, I usually say to myself, "Well, he must be having a bad day," rather than getting angry or feeling overwhelmed.

Perhaps the breathing breaks, which are essentially minimeditations, have already begun to help you in this way, easing the stress of tense interactions or monstrous tasks. Hopefully, the meditative breathing in the restorative yoga poses has also relieved some of the day's worries and returned you to your living, breathing body.

Today I want you to think about deepening and expanding the simple practices of watching your breath and maybe extending the time you practice. Why wouldn't you want to give yourself this incredible relief? Perhaps try watching your breath for 15 minutes rather than the usual 3, 5, or 10 minutes.

Before your head starts to run with the fear of another time commitment, I know you are busy, which is one of the reasons you are Spent. And I know I am already giving you many things to think about and do on a daily basis. But I guarantee that the time you spend meditating will actually create hours in the day because you will be more relaxed, focused, and energized as a result of your practice.

One of the most challenging things about most meditation practices is that they ask you to sit, which we already do too much of. How much time do you already spend sitting every day? And for those who are Spent, sitting meditation tends to add more physical stress to the chronic tension and stress we are trying to relieve.

So, unlike more traditional meditation practices, I do not recommend sitting meditation (initially, anyway) for my patients who are suffering from Spent. It just doesn't seem to help. Sure, down the road, once a patient is feeling better, sitting meditation is fine. But, in my opinion, asking someone who is tired, physically achy, and stiff and already spends too much time in a chair to increase sitting—in a chair or on a cushion—is downright cruel and does nothing for his or her health and well-being. But again, this is about my giving you options to help you find and establish your rhythm of health and well-being. If you find that sitting meditation works for you, then by all means do it.

As you know, there are many many schools, formulas, and texts for how to practice meditation. Meditation is one of those things that is very personal. For nearly every one of my patients, there is a different practice. I believe everyone has to find the one that suits his or her needs and tastes. If you already have a practice or are familiar with one that you like, make a commitment to integrate the practice more fully into your daily schedule. But if just the idea of this tires you out, try one of my techniques.

For those of you who have not enjoyed watching your breath or found it strenuous, in a few days I will teach you a nature meditation, which does not focus on breathing, but you will find that you are breathing more deeply when you are done. For now, try the technique on page 137, as it is as much of a restorative yoga pose as a meditation. No matter what you prefer, I urge you to try this method. It is incredibly effective for lightening a heavy heart and easing stress or fatigue.

The point of all meditation is to bring us back to our most essential selves—to the rhythm of the breath, our lungs, which expand and contract next to our heart.

The Pulse
○ ● ● ○ ● ● ○ ● ● ○

- **Depending upon how you feel, do 30 or 35 minutes of restorative exercise. If you are still tired, do not add the additional 5 minutes. If it is sunny out, perhaps take your walk outside.**
- ○ Continue taking a multivitamin and an adaptogenic formula.
- ○ Continue to follow the Spent restorative eating program, liberating your body from sugar, artificial sweeteners, processed foods, gluten, dairy products, alcohol, caffeinated beverages, and factory-farmed meats, poultry, and eggs.

SLEEP BEAT

- ○ Turn off your TV, cell phones, and computers by 10 p.m.
- ○ Keep your bedroom cool. Keep the thermostat low.
- ○ For uninterrupted melatonin production, darken your bedroom completely or use an eye mask.
- ○ Continue to regulate your sleep schedule.
- **Try practicing this meditation, which incorporates the Chair-Supported Savasana (page 94) before bed. Practice for 15 minutes.**

MEDITATION USING
CHAIR-SUPPORTED SAVASANA

Set an alarm clock for 17 minutes from now. This way you don't have to worry about time (I've allotted 2 minutes for you to get yourself into the pose).

Get into the Chair-Supported Savasana. If you prefer Viparita Karani (legs up the wall), you can also use this pose (page 115).

Read through the following instructions once or twice. As with the mindful breathing exercise, you don't have to memorize what to do—there is no right or wrong way to meditate. These are just guidelines to give you a sense of how to move into and try this particular type of meditation. When you feel you are ready, close your eyes and begin your version of a meditation practice.

1. *Allow your body to settle.*
2. *Scan your body, noticing where it is making contact with the floor and the chair and noticing where it is not. For instance, does the back of the left calf feel different than the back of the right? Travel from your feet up and out to your arms, and then on up to your head.*
3. *Notice if your body feels spacious or tight. More often than not, just noticing where you feel tight will bring about an autonomic response and release in that area.*
4. *Once you have scanned your body—toe to head—bring your attention to your breath, breathing in through the nose and out through the nose. Your mouth is softly closed, your jaw is easy. Notice that you are breathing in. Notice that you are breathing out. Notice that just noticing that you are breathing might change or alter the breath. Remember: there is no need to force or control the breath. Just allow your body to breathe.*
5. *Notice where the breath is going. After a minute or so, take a moment or two to watch where the breath is traveling in the body. Notice also where the breath doesn't travel to. Is it going to the chest but not the lower back?*

(continued on next page)

6. Become more and more sensitive to your breath. Become more and more in tune with where it moves on the inhale and exhale—and where it doesn't.

7. Allow your awareness of the breath to bring ease into your entire body. Your muscles and tendons are not working. Your bones are malleable. Everything is moving toward the earth, yet you feel supported and buoyant.

8. Continue watching the breath move in and out of the body in this way, noticing that you are breathing in, noticing that you are breathing out. As with mindful breathing, this is the main focus of this meditation.

9. When the alarm sounds, inhale and exhale deeply, allowing the inhale to move down to the toes and the exhale to move up and out of the tops of the shoulders. Take three more breaths like this: inhaling down, exhaling up and out. Then bend your knees into your chest and roll onto your right side. Pause there for a moment and then bring yourself up to sit. Move slowly, retaining a sense of ease and relaxation.

Note: If you are really struggling with watching your breath, you might want to try One Global Breath goggles. The goggles fit on your face like a ski mask and help direct your focus to your breath using light. The instructions are to inhale when the goggle lights turn on and exhale when they turn off. You can regulate the timing of the inhale or exhale and how long you want to practice—5, 15, or 30 minutes. I have found these goggles to be an extremely helpful way to get my patients to learn to focus on their breath.

Go to www.spentmd.com to learn more.

DAILY BEAT 21

EASE UP

It has been three weeks—perhaps a long and intense three weeks. Today is a day devoted to your easing up—physically and emotionally. Most of us are Spent because we live in overdrive. And, as you know, much of this program is about helping you find ways to ease up and chill out. Listening to music is one of the best ways I know to do this.

Human beings have been using sound and music for healing since the beginning of recorded history. In ancient Greece, Apollo was the god of both music and medicine. In the East, chanting, mantras, and "singing bowls" are used to access deeper states of consciousness and heal the body. In Africa, drumming and music are activities that are natural to everyone, music being part of all ceremonies and rituals and not necessarily for entertainment. It is a by-product of the modern era that we enjoy music as entertainment. Most cultures knew the power of music to enhance worship, aid hunting, help healing, and promote well-being.

One of my favorite stories that demonstrates the healing power of sound is about Alfred Tomatis, M.D. Dr. Thomatis is a French eye, ear, nose, and throat specialist renowned for his revolutionary research into sound. He once treated an abbey of Benedictine monks who during the mid-1960s became extremely fatigued and depressed. No one could figure out why. They tried increasing their caloric intake, adding meat to their vegetarian diet, taking vitamins and even drugs, and getting more sleep. Nothing worked, and their symptoms worsened. Dr. Tomatis traced the problem to a 1960 Vatican directive that had eliminated their traditional Gregorian chanting in favor of a "more constructive" use of their time. Dr. Tomatis's theory was that the monks' daily six hours of chanting had energized them, so they didn't need much sleep or food. Dr. Tomatis prescribed that they chant again. Nine months later, the monks were happy and healthy and had returned to their ascetic lifestyle of hard work and spare vegetarian diet. The Gregorian chanting gave them a much-needed sense of joy and self-expression to sustain their monastic lives.

Music also sustains me. When I get to work in the morning, the first thing I do is turn on the CD player. When I come home after a hard day's work, there's nothing better than sitting down and putting on some music. Music is always playing in our house. I love world music and African music in particular. Because I can't understand the words, I have to feel them through the rhythm. The sounds bypass my thinking mind, my rational mind, and touch me at a core level. As Bob Marley said, "The thing about music is that when it hits, you feel no pain."

For me, listening to music is not just a release, it is another kind of meditation. I become less in tune with my mind's inner chatter and external stimulation and more present. As with meditation, music has also helped me connect to some of my deepest feelings and self—maybe even my "soul." And as you know, music promotes an amazing sense of well-being.

In my clinical experience, I have found it wildly effective when I need help inducing this sense of well-being, teaching people to meditate, and soothing patients who are tense but need energy because they are Spent. It has also helped patients release feelings that were "stuck" in their bodies.

I have been using music and sound in my practice for the last twenty years and have seen profound results, particularly when I use it in conjunction with acupuncture. I give the patient an acupuncture treatment and while the needles are in, I put headphones on the patient and play a CD. I suggest that the patient close her eyes so that the listening becomes more acute. I then encourage her to hear with her whole body, not only to listen to the full spectrum of sounds but also to feel the vibrations of the sounds. This listening seems to amplify the effects of the acupuncture.

Sound triggers responses all over your body and affects your cellular rhythm, right down to your vibrating atoms. If you live in a city, traffic, car horns, sirens, jackhammers, airplanes, and a million variations of the human voice vibrate constantly. If you live in the supposedly quieter suburbs, leaf blowers, lawn mowers, kids at play, and barking dogs still assault your eardrums.

You can counter sound's negative effects by using it positively and deliberately: relaxing music slows heart and breathing rates and creates a feeling of well-being. Upbeat music stimulates and energizes you. But not any old music will do. If you hate classical music, for example, a Mozart sonata probably won't relax you, nor will a Stravinsky scherzo energize you. Studies show that the most profound benefits occur only when you listen to music you enjoy. So pull something out that you love and crank it up!

The Pulse

○ • • ○ • • ○ • • ○

- On your way to work, to the market, to your living room, or wherever you are headed and throughout the day, ease your pulse. Listen to some of your favorite music. Sing or hum along. Allow the joy of the music to move into you. *Note: Normally, your heart rate at rest should be at about 70 beats per minute for men and about 75 for women. Music pulsing at about 60 beats per minute (most reggae music pulses at around 60 beats per minute) is ideal for helping induce an alpha state, the same relaxed state created by meditation and biofeedback. Your body syncs with or mimics a pulse greater than your own. This is important because you use less energy when you're in sync with your surrounding energy. If you can't listen to music at work, keep music inside you physically and emotionally. If you don't have a clue what to listen to or would like some suggestions for music that will ease your pulse, I've listed two good resources on page 318. For my favorite CDs and a more extensive list of music, go to www.spentmd.com.*

- Take a day off from your restorative exercise.

SLEEP BEAT

- Bring ease to your neck and spine: try the following exercises, Occipital Release and Cats and Dogs.

OCCIPITAL RELEASE
(NECK AND CRANIAL RELEASE)

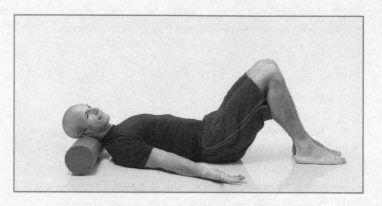

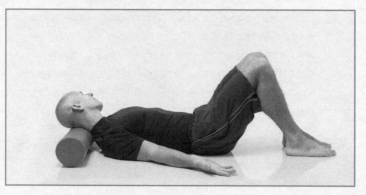

Place your foam roller behind your neck with the base of your skull resting on the roller. Release all tension in your neck by allowing the weight of your head to rest on the roller as you slowly rock your head from right to left and then left to right. Pause on each tender area and take a few deep inhales and exhales, allowing your muscles to relax into the support of the roller.

Benefits: Promotes cervical mobility, massages tight neck and head musculature, relieves headaches and sinus congestion, eases eyes tired from the computer.

Caution: Keep the range of motion comfortable as you move slowly from side to side. Avoid movement if cervical disc herniation is present.

CATS AND DOGS

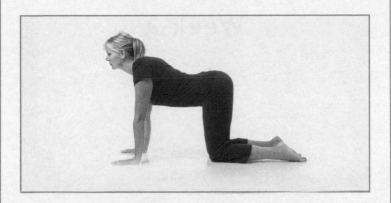

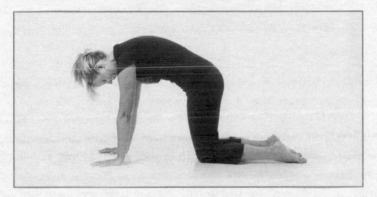

Get down on your hands and knees, making sure that your hips are balanced over your knees and your hands are directly beneath your shoulders.

Inhale, sinking your navel, front ribs, and chest toward the floor. Let your shoulder blades move together, and gaze softly upward. The front of the body opens with this inhale. As you exhale, draw in your navel, ribs, and chest, rounding them up toward the ceiling. Allow your head, neck, and tailbone to release toward the floor. Let all the air in your lungs seep out. Repeat this inhaling and exhaling sequence 5 to 10 times.

Benefits: Creates spine and hip mobility.

Caution: If your knees are sensitive, add a blanket under your shins and knees.

Week 4

Release

Some of us think holding on makes us strong; but sometimes it is letting go.

—Herman Hesse

Congratulations! You are halfway through the six-week Spent restorative program! Now that you have some more energy, it is time to go a bit deeper—to pull out and let go of some of the underlying issues and habits that can contribute to Spent, from household toxins and genetically modified foods to spending too much of your day in a chair. Yes, sitting can make you Spent. We will also look at ways to boost your newfound sense of health, ways for you to let loose and laugh and enjoy being a human being once again.

Thanks to a continuous adherence to the Spent restorative eating program—no sugar, artificial sweeteners, processed foods, gluten, dairy, caffeinated beverages, or alcohol—and restorative exercise, an adaptogenic formula, a multivitamin, new sleep habits, and restorative yoga, most of my patients feel remarkably better. So while you will continue to follow this protocol, get ready to release the old and make room for the new.

DAILY BEAT 22

STOP EATING UNFERMENTED SOY AND
GENETICALLY MODIFIED CORN

While soy and corn are less detrimental and Spent-causing than sugar or gluten, they do add to the body's burden and can throw us out of rhythm.

For the last twenty years, soy has been touted as the ultimate replacement for animal protein, fish, and dairy products. The thinking goes that Asian societies are healthier because they eat large amounts of soy. But the truth is that Asian cultures consume soy foods in small amounts (about 2 teaspoons a day) as a condiment and not as a replacement for animal foods. According to Sally Fallon and Mary Enig, Ph.D., two experts on the subject, soy foods were traditionally fermented to neutralize toxins in soybeans, whereas most modern soy foods are not fermented. They are processed in a way that denatures the proteins and increases the levels of carcinogens in the soy.[1]

A splash here, a cube of tofu there are not going to hurt you. But having soy milk or tofu many times a week may. I cannot tell you how many patients of mine I've seen whose natural rhythms have been interrupted by soy. Finally, soy phytoestrogens can disrupt endocrine function and cause thyroid dysfunction, which, when you are Spent, can be a major issue.

Corn is a problem too. Apart from the fact that corn contains a high amount of sugar and often a lot of mold, most corn you buy in the United States is genetically modified (GMO). GMO corn was lauded by farmers and biotech firms for its ability to be disease- and pest-resistant and more bountiful. Genetically modified organisms are different from hybridized plants, which are naturally occurring. An example of hybridization is one breed of dog mating with another. An example of a GMO would be mating an eggplant and a dog in a Petri dish, which is, obviously, not naturally occurring. GMOs are not good for us. We don't know the long-term health risks of ingesting this kind of biological experiment. Most countries in Europe and Japan—even in Africa—are refusing GMO grains because they have seen GMOs cause irreversible metabolic damage. The Spent restorative eating program has already taken out high-fructose corn syrup, which is often the most common way people consume GMO corn. But I strongly urge you to cut out GMO corn (and any other GMO grain, for that matter). There is really no need for it in your diet—ever, unless in small quantities and organic.

As for soy, I suggest you stop eating unfermented soy for the next three weeks. Then maybe you can reintroduce it into your diet, but in very small, supplementary amounts. If you want to eat soy products, eat tempeh, miso, natto, and wheat-free tamari (soy sauce), which have been fermented. With fermentation, these foods have had their nutrients that inhibit digestion and absorption of some minerals neutralized and can be eaten safely in small amounts. Don't rely on soy as a protein source; instead, think of it as a condiment—a small part of a balanced diet.

The Pulse
○ • • ○ • • ○ • • ○

- If you eat corn, make a commitment to stop buying GMO corn and start buying local organic corn in season and eat it only in small quantities. Again, the more consumer demand for this there is, the more available and less expensive it will be.
- To further heal from Spent, stop consuming soy for the next three weeks.
- Resume your restorative exercise practice, walking for 35 minutes today, preferably outside. Again, remember to work at a pace that is simultaneously challenging and not exhausting.
- Make a beautiful lunch for yourself today. Notice how eating colorful, organic food really does make a difference and try the Smoothie of the Week, the Greeno Mojito Avocado Smoothie (page 270). It is fresh and minty.

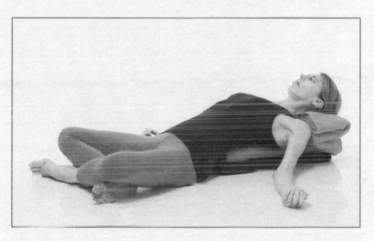

SLEEP BEAT

- Before bed, practice this restorative pose, which is a modified
  version of my favorite restorative yoga pose, Supta Baddha
  Konasana (SOOP tah BAW-dah cone-NAW-sah-nah), or God-
  dess Pose, for ten minutes. After about 5 minutes, this pose
  has a strong, beneficial effect, calming the breathing and
  soothing the emotional center of the chest. It releases stress
  and the frustrations of the day. It can be practiced after meals,
  relaxing the abdominal organs if indigestion is a problem.

MODIFIED SUPTA BADDHA KONASANA

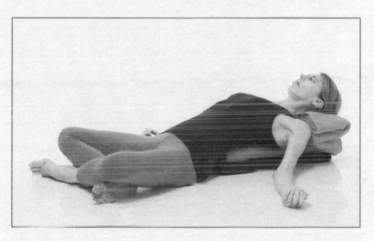

*This is where the yoga bolster I mentioned earlier really becomes useful, be-
cause it makes doing the pose much easier. However, you can use a sofa cushion or neatly folded blankets if you want to give it a try and don't have a
bolster. Sit down on the floor with your bolster and blanket nearby. Place the
bolster behind you so that it is snuggled up against your sacrum and butt.*

(continued on next page)

Take an easy cross-legged position. Don't fold your legs too tightly. Now notice in the photograph how the blankets are used to support the head. Fold your yoga blanket in half and then in thirds, so that when you lie back, your head is higher than your heart and your chin is parallel to the floor, not tipping up to the ceiling or down toward your chest. If the blanket feels too bulky, take out a fold until you find a way for your head to feel easy, with the head above the heart and the heart above your groin. As you can see in the picture, there is a natural slope from the model's forehead down to her feet. If you are like me and have tight hips and need to support your knees so that the cross-legged position is not pulling on your groin, put a cushion under each thigh.

Remember, setting up these restorative yoga poses is a skill that you learn, as are the subtleties of letting your face and throat relax as you completely rest onto the support of the bolster.

When you finally find the right position, you will feel an inner "aahh." Stay with this, watching your breath move into and out of your body for about 10 minutes. Do not force or control it; just notice that you are breathing in and breathing out.

DAILY BEAT 23

RESTORE YOUR GUT WITH PROBIOTICS

Healthy bacteria that live naturally in your gut are known as "probiotics" ("for life"). They are responsible for manufacturing key nutrients and limiting the growth of yeast and unhealthy bacteria. They're essential for digesting fruit, vegetables, and legumes, and they minimize digestive problems such as lactose intolerance and diarrhea. Two of the best-researched probiotics are *Lactobacillus* and *Bifidobacterium*.

In my experience, most people who are Spent do not have enough healthy bacteria in their guts. This can manifest itself in a number of ways—from chronic indigestion, gas, bloating, and abdominal pain to irritable bowel syndrome or other digestive disturbances (as you now know, IBS can also be a result of gluten intolerance). Most of us have unhealthily low levels because of frequent antibiotic use—often from childhood years, when we were prescribed penicillin or amoxicillin for acne, every sore throat, ear infection, and runny nose. And I discussed all the antibiotics in our commercial meats and dairy foods. These days, well-informed doctors recommend taking and replacing probiotics when a patient is taking antibiotics. But this supplementation is not enough, particularly for those who are Spent. Our digestion needs to be functioning optimally at all times so that we can absorb the nutrients we so desperately need. I want you to begin supplementing with probiotics or adding them to your smoothie. If you have serious digestive problems, I recommend looking at the Troubleshooting chapter (page 241) or, for an even more substantial discussion of digestive problems, going to www.spentmd.com.

The Pulse

○ ● ● ○ ● ● ○ ● ● ○

- Add probiotics to your morning smoothie or buy them in capsule form and take them with your smoothie. See www .spentmd.com for my favorite brands. If you are buying them at the store, look for refrigerated brands and make sure that there are at least 10 billion to 15 billion viable bacteria per serving.
- Release your feet with the Ultimate Foot Massage (page 92) before you do 35 minutes of restorative exercise.
○ Continue taking a multivitamin and an adaptogenic formula.
○ Continue to follow the Spent restorative eating program, liberating your body from sugar, artificial sweeteners, processed foods, gluten, dairy products, factory-farmed meats, soy, GMO corn, alcohol, and caffeinated beverages.
○ Take a few breathing breaks throughout the day.

SLEEP BEAT

○ Turn off your TV, cell phones, and computers by 10 p.m.
○ Keep your bedroom cool. Keep the thermostat low.
○ Darken your bedroom completely or use an eye mask.
○ To support your body's rhythms, regulate your sleep schedule.
- Soothe your belly and gut even more by doing belly breathing, either in a basic Savasana (page 75) or with your legs up the wall in Viparita Karani (page 115).

The internationally renowned yoga teacher Donna Farhi says, "Our breath is constantly rising and falling, ebbing and flowing, entering and leaving our bodies. Full-body breathing is an extraordinary symphony of both powerful and subtle movements that massage our internal organs, oscillate our joints, and alternately tone and release all the muscles in the body. It is a full participation with life." I completely agree.

Most of us breathe through our mouths into our upper chests and never allow our inhales to move through our nose down into our bellies. This kind of shallow breathing only brings more tension to your neck and shoulders, whereas breathing into the belly and down into the entire lower half of the body relaxes the stomach and diaphragm and "releases" your organs. Follow the instructions for the basic Savasana (page 75) or Viparita Karani (page 115), and when you have settled into the pose, begin inhaling into and exhaling from your belly, allowing it to contract and expand. With every exhale, allow yourself to breathe out completely and notice the spontaneous inhale that follows. Set a timer for 10 minutes. Follow these long, slow belly breaths, inhaling so that the belly rises and exhaling so that the belly falls. When you are done, notice that your lower back, shoulders, and neck feel more spacious.

DAILY BEAT 24

BE HUMAN

We are in the middle of the middle of adding and subtracting and subtracting and adding. How's it going? Are you hating it or loving it? How do you feel? A bit more energized or still tired? Hopefully, your body is feeling better, but it is likely that your mind, which, according to the yoga master B. K. S. Iyengar, is the hardest part of the body to adjust, might still be Spent.

First of all, there is your busy life, which has not stopped. Then there is the fact that this program gives you so much to work with and on. Even I, who have worked with these ideas and methods for years, noticed that my brain felt like a scrambled egg as I was putting all this down on paper. But over the years, I have also noticed another reason why my patients' minds still feel tired after their bodies have begun to heal. What seems to happen is that my patients start feeling better, and then they get so excited by this newfound energy and physical freedom that they want to do everything—including taking and using every suggestion I give them to heal from Spent.

This is completely understandable. My patients start feeling good—often for the first time in months or years—and then they want to feel incredible. Who wouldn't want to take it further? But this kind of thinking can lead you right back to Spent.

Healing from Spent is about moving toward your natural genetic human rhythms. And although part of this involves taking action—eating nourishing food when your body needs it, sleeping when it is dark, and releasing tension from your body so that it can move more freely—healing from Spent is also about learning not to use your mind as your personal drill sergeant. From the time most of us open our eyes in the morning, our brain is cruising through the list of things we have to get done, reviewing calls and e-mails and conversations had or to be had. Living with all these lists, aiming to please and perform, is a surefire way to be Spent. After all, we are human beings, not human doings.

Today, rather than running through The Pulse and checking the items off the list, listen to how you feel. What do you need? Are you feeling guilty because you haven't yet started your restorative exercise program? Or are you craving sugar, caffeine, or a particular gluten- or dairy-rich food? If you are, it is completely normal. If you have eaten your favorite candy or had half a cup of caffeinated coffee or a piece of bread, don't worry about it. The most important thing to remember at this stage is not to be too hard on yourself about relapses. If all you have had is something like one cookie, a cappuccino here and there, and a slice of cheese over the course of the last couple of weeks, you are doing incredibly well. The changes I'm asking for can, in every sense, be extraordinarily hard. You are literally reconceiving the way you eat, sleep, and live—and, most important, think.

By changing your thinking, I mean that I want you to begin doing what is good and feels good to you—not what your boss or I say. It is your body, and you know far more about it than I do. So today, if you feel as if the restorative exercise is not working and you want to go for a long run, do it and then see how you feel. Or if you are annoyed with the whole process of doing a beat per day, take a day off. If you would like to, do it all "wrong" today. Forget your multivitamin. Have too big a meal for dinner. My point is that I want you to let your process be way less than perfect. In fact, let it be messy. Throughout this program it is important to let yourself play, bringing things back in and letting them go—this is the only way you are going to find out how *you* feel, what *your* body needs, *your* true rhythm. Maybe from today's running experiment, you will discover that running does tire you out, but that will lead you to another physical activity that you've always wanted to try but haven't because you've always run. Maybe not.

The most extraordinary thing about our lives as human beings is that we are all uniquely flawed, yet we all somehow manage to live together in a beautiful collage of mass confusion and mess and survive. The more we embrace the confusion, gray areas, and uncertainty of it all, the more mental and physical ease we will have. As one of my favorite musicians, Michael

Franti, says, "Don't let mistakes be so monumental, don't let your love be so confidential, don't let your mind be so darn judgmental, and please let your heart be more influential."

The Pulse

○ • • ○ • • ○ • • ○

- Take the day off or stay on the program. Play. The following beats are just suggestions.
○ Continue adding probiotics to your morning smoothie or taking them with it.
○ Do 35 minutes of restorative exercise with a friend.
○ If you are still struggling with taking breathing breaks, you are not alone. It takes some people years to get good at it. For help go to www.spentmd.com for easy instructions for the One Global Breath Meditation.

SLEEP BEAT

- Maybe before bed, to ease spinal tension, do 10 Cats and Dogs (page 143) and then practice the Modified Supta Baddha Konasana restorative pose (page 147) for 10 minutes. *Note:* As you get into the pose, notice which way you "naturally" cross your legs and switch the cross so that you are crossing them in an unhabitual pattern. Notice how different it feels—just another way for us to feel how our body is different on one side from the other.

DAILY BEAT 25

FIGHT CHAIR BODY

All of us are victims of the chair. I have found that most of my patients who are suffering from Spent spend far too much time sitting, which is perhaps the worst position for our body's mechanics. The lower back becomes sore and irritated from all the tail tucking, the shoulders are encouraged to hunch and slump, and, worst of all, our hips lock up. Tight hips often lead to more severe lower back injuries, as well as knee and shoulder problems. Why? If our hips don't move the way they are supposed to, the stress travels down and up the body to areas that can absorb and flex. For instance, if your hips are tight and you play tennis regularly, your flexible knees and ankles will have to compensate for the inflexibility of the hips. Over time, this overuse and overstretching will create a knee and/or ankle problem.

What's worse is that sitting actually atrophies our walking muscles. Our crucial core muscles—the ones that support our posture, organs, continence, and sexual health—also weaken. The consequence of these weak and unhealthy muscles is much like our tennis example. The more flexible areas (especially the spine) and the extremities have to take on more stress and use. Lower back pain, neck pain, carpal tunnel syndrome, and knee pain can often be traced back to sitting. Sitting too much changes our natural posture, joint mechanics, and ability to use the muscles of the back, butt, and thighs. This forces smaller muscles and joints to perform tasks that really should be done by these bigger muscles and joints.

To combat chair body, let me give you two excellent exercises to begin playing with. These exercises, paired with Spinal Reset (page 81) and the Neck and Shoulder Release Using a Foam Roller (page 125) I've already taught you, are the ultimate recipe for a tired, sore back. You can do these several times a day at your office. Just bring a tennis ball to work and take a few minutes every few hours to relieve your body of the shape of the chair.

Beyond these exercises, the greatest opponent of the chair is movement. No matter what you do for a living, think about ways you can bring more movement into your life. If you are a computer programmer or film editor or work in any other profession where you log hours at a time in a chair, try to take a seven-minute bathroom break every hour or two. On this break, walk around. Walk up and down some stairs. Swing your arms as you walk down the hall. Take fifteen or twenty steps as though you were in a marching band, bringing the knees high up. Go outside and walk around the building's parking lot or walk around the building or house or block. When it comes to fighting the chair, these little breaks are potent healers. They get us breathing and the blood moving again, which helps keep us energized and in rhythm.

Don't let the chair win. Fight back!

The Pulse

○ • • ○ • • ○ • • ○

- Beyond your 35 minutes of restorative exercise, find more ways to move. Take the stairs. Walk to the market. Walk around the block or your office building (this will also increase your sun time!).
○ To support healthy digestive function, continue adding probiotics to your morning smoothie, or take them with it.

SLEEP BEAT

○ Stay on your new sleep schedule.
- Try some chair-fighting technology (page 157) before you go to bed. Muscle tension is one of the most common ways of holding emotions in. And our hips—probably because they protect our sexual organs—seem to be the place where many of us store feelings. This tension can result in lower back pain,

sciatica, and very tight hips. As you know, the less tension there is in the fascia, the less Spent we are. So try these hip releases to prepare for bed.

HIP AND BACK RELEASE

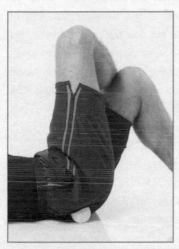

Lie on your back on a firm surface (a wood floor is best). Place two tennis balls in the center of the back of your pelvis, ensuring that they sit on muscle (what would be the "dimple" of your gluteal muscles if you were a body-builder) and not the sacral bone. The tennis balls should be 2 to 4 inches apart and 2 to 4 inches below the top of your pelvis. Cross your right leg over your left and then allow your right knee to open to the right, taking your body weight with it. Slowly massage your right glute over the tennis ball, searching for tender spots. Hold on each tender area for 1 minute, then move on to a new area. Switch sides and massage the left glute.

Benefits: Releases locked glutes from sitting. The release increases blood flow to hip musculature and reduces glute-induced back strain. It also mobilizes hips and low back.

Caution: Avoid if you experience sharp pain or are in the acute stage of sciatica. Keep the range of motion small if you have had a hip replacement.

PIRIFORMIS STRETCH

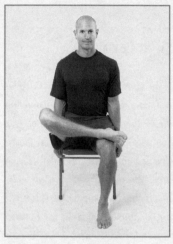

Sit toward the front of a chair seat so that the edge just hits the intersection of your butt muscles and hamstrings. Cross your right ankle over the left knee so that the ankle bone rests on the soft flesh just above the knee. Flex the right foot. Lengthen your spine, making the sides of your body longer, and then lean slightly forward with this extended spine. Breathe deeply. You should feel the stretch deep in your butt muscles. Hold for 1 to 2 minutes, moving the torso closer to the legs as the hip opens. Switch sides.

Benefits: *Mobilizes the hips. Reduces strain on the lower back caused by tight hips. Excellent for lower back pain, tight hips, piriformis syndrome, and sciatica.*

Caution: *Avoid rounding the spine; keep the back flat and lean forward from the hips.*

DAILY BEAT 26

LIMIT YOUR EXPOSURE TO CHEMICALS

Baby boomers will remember the slogan "Better living through chemistry." It was part of a campaign that started some sixty years or so ago, when chemical companies and other major industries began indoctrinating us into believing that synthetics (processed, packaged, junk, and fake foods; coatings, pesticides, and pharmaceuticals) were better and more effective than naturally occurring products, foods, and medicines.

As a result, over the ensuing years we've introduced thousands of chemicals into our food, air, and water without knowing how they'll react in our bodies or what their synergistic effects might be. "Synergistic" means that the total effect of two or more chemicals is greater than the sum of their individual effects.

I've already mentioned the fact that we eat foods depleted of essential nutrients, which are replaced by GMOs and chemical additives in processed foods. These act synergistically with the synthetic chemicals that we absorb through our skin or inhale from the air, which compounds our body burden, throwing us even further out of rhythm.

Most of us believe that environmental toxins are evident to the senses. This is completely false. There are thousands of extremely hazardous toxins that you cannot see, smell, taste, or necessarily feel. And you are exposed to these pollutants in many combinations. For instance, now that you are paying more attention to what you are putting into your body, it's time to start thinking about what you are putting around your body: the water you bathe in, the air you breathe, the products you clean your house with.

More and more research now suggests that environmental pollutants disrupt our hormonal systems, sending mixed or unclear messages to their targets. Many of the chemicals dumped into our environment have been banned in Europe but are still in wide use in the United States. According to several studies, they are, in reality, low-level poisons that slowly erode the functioning of our hormones and contribute to feeling Spent—particularly the chemicals we use to "treat" and "clean" our water with.[2,3,4]

I believe, as do many environmental experts, that two of the greatest threats to our thyroid gland, a key hormonal system, are fluoride and chlorine, which are both in our water supply.[5] Fluoride is also in our toothpaste, and chlorine is in many household cleaners, though it is often described as "sodium hypochlorite" or "hypochlorite." Liquid household bleaches are approximately 5% sodium hypochlorite solutions. The basis of this belief is that both chlorine and fluoride are chemically related to iodine, which is an essential component in the synthesis of thyroid hormone. They block iodine receptors, interfering with iodine metabolism, and therefore impair thyroid function.

First, let's take a quick look at fluoride. Adding fluoride to our drinking water is widely accepted, but I agree with the many concerned physicians and scientists such as Robert Carlton, Ph.D., a former EPA scientist, who question the wisdom and safety of this massive public health initiative.[6,7]

The short-range goal of reducing tooth decay seems to have blinded us to the long-range risks fluoridation subjects people to. If you ask me, fluoridated municipal water supplies may well be a reason why thyroid dysfunction is so common. Fluoride's ability to impair thyroid function is perhaps best illustrated by the fact that up until the 1970s European doctors used fluoride as a thyroid-suppressing medication for patients with an overactive thyroid. If you'd like to learn more about the potential risks of adding fluoride to our water systems, visit www.fluoridealert.org.

Here's another fluoride fact: drinking large amounts of green tea and black tea may also be sources of fluoride exposure, because the tea plant (*Camilla sinensis*) is known to pull a high amount of fluoride from the soil. As noted, fluoride is toxic to the thyroid, which may outweigh any of tea's benefits for people who are Spent. Having said that, having a cup or two of tea a day probably poses no problems.

As for chlorine, the Environmental Protection Agency says that most human exposure to chlorine actually occurs during its industrial use, not through laundry bleach or swimming pool chemicals, but the fact is that even at low levels, chlorine causes environmental and bodily harm. It may take years before we fully comprehend the health consequences of the

23 billion pounds of the stuff that are produced in this country every year. Here's what we do know: exposure to chlorine affects the immune system, blood, heart, and respiratory system of animals. And I believe it contributes to Spent because it's a toxin that impairs the function of your thyroid gland as well.

This is why I *insist* that you get a water filter, at least for your drinking water. Of course, a home water filtration system is even better. See Resources (page 305) or go to www.spentmd.com or www.custompure.com for more information.

Though you'd think that any chemical used commercially would be thoroughly tested for safety, you'd be wrong. The National Resource Defense Council says that the majority of the more than two thousand chemicals that come onto the market every year don't undergo even the simplest toxicity tests.

Unfortunately, it could be several generations before we fully comprehend the impact these toxins have on our bodies. I'm convinced that there's a link between the epidemic of Spent I'm witnessing among my patients and the proliferation of toxic chemicals like chlorine and fluoride in our environment.

The good news is that there are some easy and economical ways to limit the amount of toxins that attack our system.

A FEW SIMPLE RULES
FOR CLEANER LIVING

Don't wear shoes in the house. Go barefoot or wear slippers—most dirt, pesticides, and lead come in on your shoes.

Place floor mats by your entryways. This way more dirt and residue from your shoes will stay on the mat.

Be conscious of the potential of wall-to-wall carpeting to hold toxins. If possible, replace your wall-to-wall carpeting with hardwood floors, all-natural linoleum, or ceramic tiles. Most wall-to-wall carpeting off-gases toxic fumes that can add to your body's burden. If you must have it, use nontoxic glues, adhesives, stains, or sealers for installation. But know that natural-fiber wool and cotton rugs are best.

Keep the air clean. Have your air ducts and vents cleaned with nontoxic cleaners. Get a portable air cleaner/purifier, especially for bedrooms. Use green plants as natural air detoxifiers, add fragrance with fresh flowers or herbs, and remove odors with baking soda. Keep house dust to a minimum—more dust means more toxins.

Get a shower filter. Many contaminants in tap water become gases at room temperature. A shower filter can help keep these toxins from becoming airborne.

Tell your dry cleaner not to use plastic wrap. Plastic traps the dry-cleaning chemicals on clothes and in your closet. Let your dry cleaning air out (preferably outside) before storing it. Use "wet cleaning" if you are lucky enough to have it in your area.

Avoid excess moisture and mold. Check areas—particularly your basement, kitchen, and bathrooms—for moisture accumulation and leaks. Regularly clean surfaces where mold usually grows—around showers and tubs and beneath sinks.

Switch from standard cleaning products to natural ones or make your own. See Resources on page 305 or my website, www .spentmd.com, for the products I recommend and a more complete list of ways to decrease your household toxic load.

Of course, I don't expect you to spend your evening ripping up carpeting or installing a new home water filtration system, but I do want you to begin taking steps to detoxify your home. Simple tasks such as buying a water filter for your drinking water and replacing your cleaning products with all-natural ones can make an enormous difference in your body's toxic load.

The Pulse

○ ● ● ○ ● ● ○ ● ● ○

- Buy a water filter for your drinking water and switch your household products to more body-friendly ones.
○ Do 35 minutes of restorative exercise. If you can, do it outside.
○ Continue adding probiotics to your morning smoothie or taking them with it.
○ Continue taking a multivitamin and an adaptogenic formula.
- Continue playing with your rhythm of eating. Try a new recipe from the back of the book for your lunch or dinner today.

SLEEP BEAT

○ Keep your bedroom cool. Keep the thermostat low.
○ Darken your bedroom completely or use an eye mask.
● To prepare for sleep, practice the two hip releases you learned last night (pages 157–58) and then add this third hip release technique, on the following page, which opens the front of your groin.

STANDING HIP FLEXOR STRETCH

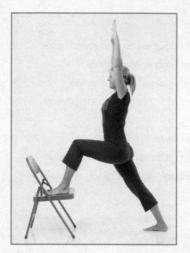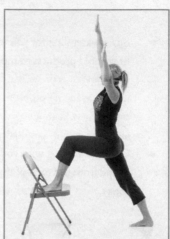

Stand in front of a straight-backed chair. Step your left foot onto the seat of the chair and move it forward until it's in the middle (prevents the chair from tipping over). Then walk your right leg back a bit, until you're in a long lunge position. Make sure that you are far enough back that your left knee doesn't bend past your left ankle toward your toes. (If you're having trouble balancing, place the chair beside a wall so you can hang on for balance.) Now squeeze your butt muscles (glutes) and imagine your tailbone tipping and dropping down, between your legs.

Reach your arms up to the sky. Stay as tall as you can and stretch your torso to the left (toward the side of the bent front leg). You should feel a stretch across the front of your right groin. Take a few deep breaths and then bring your arms down. Repeat, moving into and out of the bend 5 times before switching sides.

Benefits: *Relieves lower back discomfort, strengthens the butt, back, and thigh muscles, opens the respiratory muscles around the rib cage and spine, improves posture and balance.*

DAILY BEAT 27

EAT SEASONALLY

Despite the fact that many of us do not live according to the seasons, our bodies still do. In the late summer and fall, our hunter and gatherer genes still prepare for the upcoming famine, which is winter. Your genes still operate under the assumption that healthy carbohydrates like vegetables and fruit are going to be scarce. So your body starts storing these carbs to see you through. For our ancestors, the long days of summer meant eating more carbohydrates to prepare. They fattened up so that they had energy to burn in the winter. But today there is no real winter. Sure, there may be snow outside, but there are still pears and apples at the market. The problem is that our body is not built to eat these carbs year-round. It is programmed to eat for winter—meat, nuts, and root vegetables, which were traditionally available—and summer—broccoli, strawberries, and tomatoes.

We are part of this universe, down to every cell. And there are universal laws that we need to abide by to stay in rhythm with nature and our nature. If we don't keep these beats, we feel off balance; sometimes we become Spent. Anything that helps us get back to nature's beat lets us feel less Spent. All of our survival mechanisms, developed over millennia on this planet, were adaptations to go with this flow of nature. Now we need to get back to adjusting to the seasons. We should try eating what is in season. Birds do it. Bears do it. In fact, other than our domesticated animals and livestock, we are the only living beings on this planet that don't eat seasonally.

I am not suggesting that you forgo salads for six months of the year, but I do think that eating more complex carbohydrates in the summer and more animal protein, nuts, and root vegetables in the winter is a good idea—especially in cold climates. As explained in the phytonutrient discussion way back in the first week, in-season vegetables tell our bodies on a cellular level how to adjust and move with the season's rhythms.

As you walk through your local market, pay attention to what is in season. When you see a "locally grown" sign, you can be sure that apples, strawberries, potatoes, squash, watermelon, and other fruits and vegetables are in season. By the way, buying local is always a good idea—not only are you supporting your local farmer, but you are also getting food that is from the earth close to where you live. You're in tune with the seasons, and the phytonutrients will be even more in tune with your needs.

Eating seasonally means constantly adding new colors, flavors, and variety to your diet. What could be better?

The Pulse
○ ● ● ○ ● ● ○ ● ● ○

- Celebrate the season with friends.
- Go to the market and plan a dinner around the season. If it is summer, make a huge salad with tomatoes, cucumbers, and all kinds of delicious summer fruits and vegetables. If it is fall, make a butternut squash soup. If it is winter, have some grass-fed meat and roasted root vegetables. If it is spring, make a salad of fresh peas, mint, and feta on a bed of baby greens.
- Take your exercise pulse and adjust accordingly. You've been practicing restorative exercise for two weeks now. How is it feeling? Are you tired by it? Or is it not feeling like enough? Do you need to do more? Take a day off if you need to or just feel like it.
○ Do the Wall Stretch (page 72) to wake up and open up your body.
○ Continue to follow the Spent restorative eating program, liberating your body from sugar, artificial sweeteners, processed foods, gluten, dairy products, factory-farmed meats, soy, GMO corn, alcohol, and caffeinated beverages.

SLEEP BEAT

○ Turn off your TV, cell phones, and computers by 10 p.m.
○ Stay on your new sleep schedule.
● If you feel like it, practice all three hip releases on pages 157, 158, and 164 before bed.
● Begin taking a Spent sleep formula.

At night, I recommend that people take nutrients that calm the body and mind down, to get ready for sleep. Go to www .spentmd.com for my favorite sleep formulas, or look for a formula that has some of the following calming amino acids: L-theanine (100 to 300 milligrams), 5-HTP (50 to 100 milligrams), gamma-aminobutyric acid (GABA) (200 to 500 milligrams), and possibly lemon balm (*Melissa officinalis*), which also has a sedative effect. Taking the minerals calcium and magnesium at night is also helpful.

DAILY BEAT 28

LAUGH

If I had no sense of humor, I would long ago have committed suicide.

—Gandhi

All of us take ourselves far too seriously, and I am as guilty as the next person. A sense of humor helps us stand back and see our selves objectively— our nuances, beliefs, tastes, idiosyncrasies, and behaviors. When we really look, it is hard to take ourselves so seriously.

Beyond giving us an often much-needed perspective, laughter helps us breathe deeply, uses our core muscles, massages the inner organs, boosts the immune system, releases endorphins (more powerful than morphine), and relieves pain. And when we are stressed and Spent, it is as important to laugh as it is to sleep.

Not only do we need to laugh at ourselves, we need to laugh with others—watching funny movies, hanging out with children, listening to a friend tell jokes. As you know, a working day filled with laughter is much shorter. My wife and I have a ritual of watching TiVoed episodes of Jon Stewart and Stephen Colbert every evening after dinner. They always make us laugh, and I find it a great way to unwind at the end of the day. But of course, what makes us laugh is not always what tickles others. Choose what makes you really laugh.

I must confess that I am having a hard time being earnest about the power of laughter. Besides, you already know how you feel when you laugh: good.

The Pulse

○ ● ● ○ ● ● ○ ● ● ○

- Find a way to bring more laughter into your day.
- Increase your restorative exercise to 40 minutes—if you feel up to it.
- Get 30 minutes of sun today.
- Take five. Before you rush out the door, sit for 5 minutes and watch your breath.
- ○ If you are still struggling with this and haven't tried our online tool, One Global Breath Meditation, go to www.spentmd .com and try it now.

SLEEP BEAT

- ○ Take the Spent sleep formula.
- Watch a funny movie (before 10 p.m.!) or read a funny book.

Week 5

Balance

To understand yourself is the beginning of wisdom.

—Krishnamurti

Following a program like the Spent restorative program is a balancing act: to do, but not to overdo.

This week focuses on helping you find your balance—in your Spent restorative eating program, in your body, and in your life. Until now we have focused on the gross imbalances in your body, which were the result of a poor diet, not enough sleep, and improper use of your body—from too much exercise to too much sitting.

In week five, I like to bring the attention to the core, the physical center of the body, and to the more subtle things that can affect a person's health—particularly the spirit. If a patient is emotionally Spent, he or she can be doing nearly everything right—a healthy diet, reasonable exercise, enough sleep—and still feel awful. Though I am not a therapist, I do talk to my patients about their lives. You may be surprised to know that even one big resentment or persistent negative train of thought can be the barricade between feeling Spent and feeling wonderful.

This week we will work on strengthening core muscles, improving hormonal function, and making sure that your cells are not being poisoned by harmful metals.

When your physical and emotional center is strong, you have the foundation for lasting health.

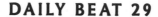

DAILY BEAT 29

EAT LOW-MERCURY FISH

Thanks to modern dentistry, most people know that mercury is toxic to humans. What most people don't know is that our greatest danger for mercury poisoning is no longer in our amalgam fillings, it is in the fish we eat. In the last ten or so years, I have found that many of my patients who eat fish regularly and are feeling Spent have high mercury levels. These levels usually decrease when they stop eating fish. In fact, I am beginning to believe that eating certain types of fish too frequently and the associated mercury toxicity may be one of the underlying factors in why so many people are feeling Spent.

Mercury poisons some of the enzymes that our body needs for cellular energy production. It also competes with essential minerals such as magnesium, zinc, and selenium. This disruption leads to a depletion of these minerals and compounds as well as our ability to produce energy in our cells. When our cells are not fed these enzymes and minerals, we no longer have energy. We become tired, develop joint and muscle pain, and have trouble sleeping, symptoms of both mercury poisoning and Spent.

Of course, this deprivation and increased toxicity can lead to all sorts of more severe health problems such as Alzheimer's disease as well. The nervous system is particularly sensitive to mercury toxicity, which is why I think it is important to be careful of what fish you eat. I must confess that I hate telling you to be wary of fish because fish is the ideal food for Spent, because of its healthy oils and protein. But now fish is, more often than not, contaminated with mercury. The fact that one of the healthiest foods has become a problem is just another sign of how profoundly we have poisoned our environment.

Here is what has happened. Coal-fired power plants release mercury into the atmosphere, and this settles in our oceans and rivers. Plants known as plankton absorb the mercury in the polluted water. Small fish then feed on the plankton. Then the larger fish eat the smaller fish that have eaten the mercury-rich plants, accumulating mercury in their tissues. The older and larger the fish, the greater the potential for high mercury levels in their bodies, which is why I suggest that you stay away from big fish such as tuna and swordfish. When you eat fish, you absorb more than 95 percent of the methyl mercury that is present in the fish and store it in your tissue. Eating smaller fish with low mercury levels is essential.

Farm-raised fish are not any healthier. In fact, in a study published in the journal *Science* in 2004, researchers discovered that farm-raised salmon had more dioxins and other chemicals such as polychlorinated biphenyls (PCBs), which the U.S. Department of Health and Human Services has determined are carcinogens, than wild salmon had.

My Guidelines on Fish

EAT AS MUCH AS YOU LIKE

Anchovies	Wild salmon (fresh and canned)
Black cod (sablefish)	Sardines (canned)

DON'T EAT MORE THAN 3 TO 4 TIMES A WEEK

Striped bass	Smoked king salmon
Catfish	Scallops
Char	Shrimp (domestic)
Clams	Pacific sole
Blue crab (mid-Atlantic)	Squid (calamari)
Croaker	Sturgeon
Flounder	Tilapia
Haddock	Rainbow trout
Mussels	Canned "chunk" or light tuna
Oysters	

DON'T EAT MORE THAN 3 TO 4 TIMES A MONTH

Bluefish

Cod

Crab

Grouper (wild)

Herring

Lobster (Maine)

Mahimahi

Pollack

Canned albacore or white tuna

Whitefish

EAT RARELY

Largemouth bass

Sea bass

White croaker

Halibut

King mackerel

Marlin

Gulf Coast oysters

Pike

Shark

Swordfish

Tilefish

Tuna steaks

Walleye

For more info, go to www.ewg.org/safefishlist.

The Pulse

○ • • ○ • • ○ • • ○

- • Commit to eating fish that is low in mercury.
- ○ Do 40 minutes of restorative exercise, being mindful of how your body feels.
- • Continue adding probiotics to this week's Smoothie of the Week, the Pineapple Peach Banana Smoothie (page 271).
- ○ Continue taking a multivitamin and an adaptogenic formula.
- • Continue playing with your rhythm of eating. Maybe make a meal using a low-mercury fish such as wild salmon.

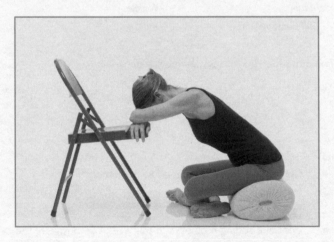

SLEEP BEAT

○ Keep your bedroom cool. Keep the thermostat low.
○ Stay on your new sleep schedule.
○ Take the Spent sleep formula.
● **Before bed, practice this forward bend using a chair and a bolster.** This pose soothes the back and eases the hips. Although it doesn't look as if you are doing much, supporting your forehead in this way calms the nervous system, and I have found this pose to be a surefire stress reliever.

CHAIR FORWARD BEND

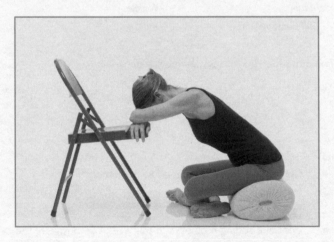

Sit on a bolster or some folded blankets, fold your arms on a chair, and rest your head on them quietly, as if you were going to sleep. Stay in the pose for 5 to 10 minutes, reversing the way your legs are crossed and your arms are folded halfway through.

DAILY BEAT 30

TAKE OMEGA-3 FISH OIL

Because we need to be careful of fish due to mercury, I recommend taking fish oil supplements (which have been checked for mercury) or flaxseed oil. These supplements will help you obtain the essential omega-3 fatty acids found in fish. Unlike trans fats, these oils lower your risk of heart disease and also lessen the inflammation that leads to a host of chronic diseases, including type 2 diabetes and arthritis. Information on omega-3s is readily available, so I will keep this overview short. Essentially, studies show that supplementing with the proper fish oil improves depression, anxiety, and fatigue and protects against heart disease, prostate cancer, and a host of other chronic illnesses. It is an essential nutrient in any weight loss program or other program to improve your general health and well-being. All of these symptoms and afflictions are associated one way or another with being Spent. This is important: do not skimp on the fish oil. Almost everyone I see needs more of these healthy omega-3 fatty acids, which become depleted when we eat too many trans fats.

Researchers have also found that certain key lipids, such as omega-3s, can improve and maintain the fluidity of cell membranes, which aids in nutrient absorption and increased energy production. In other words, when we don't have enough omega-3 fatty acids, our cell walls take up the wrong type of fat, which then affects cellular function and leads to cellular fatigue. We'll talk about this specific fatigue in a few days. For now, add omega-3s to your diet.

The Pulse
○ ● ● ○ ● ● ○ ● ● ○

- Add 1 to 2 grams of fish oil concentrate (easily available in capsule form) or 1 to 2 tablespoons of flaxseed oil to your diet

daily. Always make sure the fish oils have been tested for
mercury. See www.spentmd.com for the brands I
recommend.

O Do 40 minutes of restorative exercise—outside, if possible.

O Continue to follow the Spent restorative eating program, liberating your body from sugar, artificial sweeteners, processed
foods, gluten, dairy products, factory-farmed meats, soy,
GMO corn, mercury-laden fish, alcohol, and caffeinated
beverages.

O Listen to some of your favorite music on your way to work,
while you work, while you work out, or while cooking dinner.

SLEEP BEAT

O Turn off your TV, cell phones, and computers by 10 p.m. to
eliminate EMF radiation and brain stimulation.

O Darken your bedroom completely or use an eye mask.

O Stay on your new sleep schedule.

O Take the Spent sleep formula to calm down your nervous
system.

● **To prepare for sleep, return to your breath. Practice watching
your breath in any of your favorite restorative yoga poses, or, if
you prefer, sit in a chair or on a cushion. Notice that you are
breathing in and out through your nose. Bringing awareness
to the breath and slowing it down is an invaluable way to prepare the body to rest.** Savasana (page 75), Chair-Supported
Savasana (page 94), Supported Savasana (page 105), Viparita
Karani (page 115), and the Modified Supta Baddha Konasana
(page 147) are all wonderful positions to try this in.

DAILY BEAT 31

THINK AGAIN

If our minds are cluttered with plans, concerns, thoughts, and emotional patterns, we have no space for our true selves.

—Tulku Thondup

We have talked about many of the dietary and chemical stressors that can lead to Spent. Now it's time to focus on the organ that's intimately connected to your ability to live a happy, energetic life: your mind.

The "foods" you feed your mind are the thoughts you allow yourself to think and the subjects you allow your mind to dwell upon. If your thoughts are largely negative, if you're mired in a depressing mental swamp, or if there's a serious problem at work or at home, unless you're a really resilient person, you can end up feeling Spent.

You may not be able to change your surrounding environment, but you *can* change how you allow your environment to affect your mind. It's not as easy as it sounds, but with practice, "thinking again" can actually ease your level of mental stress. Once you get into the habit of positive thinking, you'll stop allowing your mind to dwell on thoughts that aren't positive, constructive, optimistic, and happy.

Much of what we see as "the way things are" is really just the way we choose to see them. It all depends on the lens through which you view your reality—and here's the good news: you can choose what lens to use. How you look at a situation determines whether you'll respond to it as upsetting or not.

Because our perceptions define our experience, each of us finds different and unique meaning in our world. In every moment, we have the opportunity to see things in a different way. Seeing an experience through another lens (or frame) can give us hope and a better perspective of ourselves and others. In psychology, this is called "reframing." In my world, I like to ask my patients to "think again."

If you have a negative thought—my boss sucks, my back hurts, I can't do this all today—try to think about the situation in a different way. I really like what the yogis have to say about this. In Patanjali's *Yoga Sutras* it says, "When having a negative thought or reaction, do the opposite response." In other words, change your mind.

If you're a parent, you already know about changing a mind. For instance, your child falls while trying to learn to walk; she gives you a look, checking out your face for how to react. If you rush over to her with a worried expression, she will worry too. But if you casually walk over, scoop her up, and smile, she will smile with you. You have changed her thinking about the fall so it is something that is normal and no big deal.

Changing our thinking is an important tool when we are suffering from Spent. If you see the world as a negative place, you'll only build on and enhance the discomfort your Spent symptoms cause you. The more you view events and experiences in a positive light, the more you'll heal. For instance, something good is hidden even within this challenge of being Spent. Start seeing Spent as:

- *A challenge or a growth experience, not a problem*
- *A wake-up call to reevaluate the way you want to live the rest of your life*

Spent is not a death sentence. You will get well, and you will be a lot more informed about your health and well-being after this.

Negative thoughts of powerlessness, dejection, failure, and despair reinforce and worsen Spent symptoms, whereas positive thoughts, seeing the glass half full and finding a silver lining in whatever has happened—getting fired, a breakup, a tense situation with a child—heal us. You don't need time to have perspective, just a willingness to have it.

The Pulse
○ ● ● ○ ● ● ○ ● ● ○

- Take a day off from your restorative exercise. If your body feels cranky and you feel that you must move, perhaps do a few hip releases (pages 157 and 164) and the two shoulder releases (pages 57 and 125).

- If you feel like spending time with someone, call a friend and invite him or her to dinner.
○ Continue taking a multivitamin, an adaptogenic formula, and flaxseed or fish oil.
- Make a colorful meal. Maybe just for yourself. Maybe for a friend. Maybe for your entire family.

SLEEP BEAT

○ Take the Spent sleep formula.
- To ease the spine before sleep, do 20 or so very slow Cats and Dogs (page 143), making sure to inhale deeply as you arch your back and exhale slowly as your curl your spine up to the ceiling. If you want, on the inhale you can say to yourself, "Let" and on the exhale, "Go." This is yet another way to help the mind learn to think again. After you have warmed your spine up with Cats and Dogs, do the Spinal Reset (page 81). These two exercises make a wonderful pair. And for the trifecta, add the Occipital Release (see page 142).

DAILY BEAT 32

STRENGTHEN YOUR CORE

We have already explored posture; now it's time to dive deeper, to go to your core.

Your core muscles are the foundation of your body's power. They are the foundation of deep respiration as well as of the movements of your arms and legs. These muscles lie deep within the torso and attach to the spine, the pelvis, and the muscles that support the shoulder blades. When they contract, they stabilize your spine, pelvis, and shoulders and create a solid pillar of support for the rest of your body. The stronger and more flexible your core muscles are, the easier it is for other parts of your body to operate at peak efficiency and utilize less energy.

When you're Spent, it's essential to have a strong core. Someone who is Spent needs to maximize the body's function in every way possible. Having a strong core also helps prevent injury by making us more coordinated. Core training's biggest benefit is helping you develop a level of functional fitness that makes daily living easy, enjoyable, and less draining. And training your core muscles also helps correct postural imbalances that can lead to injuries.

Most people's core muscles are weak from disuse, which can lead to chronic posture problems. Over time, bad posture damages spinal ligaments and causes disc injuries, which trigger back pain. But if you think that developing strong core muscles means doing lots of sit-ups and back extensions, think again.

When you practice my core exercises correctly, you won't feel pain, muscle burn, or even fatigue. You will feel a new sense of awareness of how your body moves and how you can improve your energy through this awareness and muscle retraining.

The simplest and most natural way to access your core muscles is through deep, rhythmic breathing. Both the belly breathing and Cats and Dogs exercises access these muscles. Learning to engage the deepest layer of abdominals with the breath helps disengage our overly developed sur-face muscles and allows the deepest layers to do their job. Core strength helps you breathe deeply, which is an essential function for oxygenating your body and helping you relax.

While you are doing these exercises, I want you to focus on the qual-ity of the movement. Go slowly, breathe deeply, and perform only as many exercises as you can with good form. If you tire, you'll find that just a few repetitions of each exercise, along with deep rib cage breathing, will help renew your energy and calm your nerves.

Note: Beyond the foam roller you ordered, balance boards and Swiss balls are great tools for core training as well as for teaching you to maintain balance and stability, both of which diminish as you age. There are a multi-tude of Web sites that offer both these tools (see Resources).

The Pulse

○ ● ● ○ ● ● ○ ● ● ○

○ Do 40 minutes of restorative exercise, remembering to alter-nate high- and low-intensity periods.

○ Continue taking flaxseed or fish oil to replenish your essential fatty acids.

○ Remember to make lunch your biggest meal. If you have been eating the same thing day after day, try some new recipes. Switch around. Diversity heals.

SLEEP BEAT

○ Darken your bedroom completely or use an eye mask.

● **Establish a regular sleep schedule.**

● **Try these three core-strengthening exercises before bed.** These simple exercises will allow you to begin to find and engage your core muscles. Ideally, I'd like for you to practice at least one of these every day for the next few weeks. You will be amazed by how quickly your core comes back. Your body *wants* to use these muscles, as they make movement much more efficient and easy!

CROSS CRAWL ON FOAM ROLLER

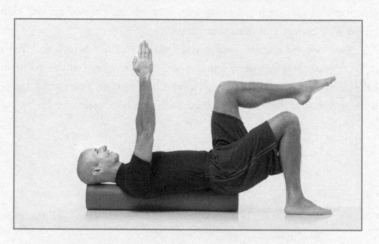

As with the Spinal Reset, lie lengthwise on the foam roller. Place your feet parallel, flat on the floor, hip width apart so that your knees line up with your hip bones and feet are directly under knees. Relax your arms at your sides, palms facing up. Slowly lift your left foot off the floor, moving your left knee over your left hip (your knee is bent), while simultaneously lifting your right hand from the floor toward the ceiling. Keep the roller as still as possible, without strain or tension, breathing deeply. Hold for several breaths, then switch sides. Perform 5 sets.

__Benefits:__ Strengthens your core muscles, improves balance, challenges coordination, reduces any physical disparity between right and left sides, which we became aware of in our Posture Check on the Floor (see page 79).

__Caution:__ If your balance is challenged, start with lifting one foot only, keeping your hands on the floor. Place a small towel under the back of your head if your neck is uncomfortable.

HIP BRIDGE WITH CACTUS ARMS

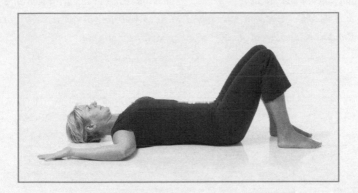

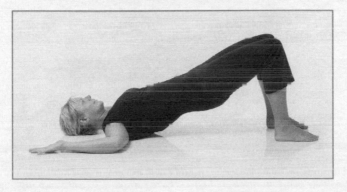

Lie on the floor with your knees bent and feet parallel and hip width apart. You arms are beside your body, either straight to the sides in a "T" or out to the sides with the elbows bent at 90 degrees with the palms facing up, in a "cactus" position (as shown in the photos). Pressing your elbows into the floor, lift your hips as high as you can. Hold for two breaths, inhaling and exhaling twice. Then slowly, gently roll your spine back to the floor, sequentially articulating each vertebra from the top to the bottom and keeping the backs of the elbows in contact with the floor. Repeat 5 times.

Benefits: Strengthens the hip extensors to open tight hip flexors, spine extensors, and core support musculature. Another chair-fighting technique!

(continued on next page)

Caution: Keep the front of your rib cage "closed" so that your ribs do not pop out and lift away from your spine or move out of line with your hips and shoulders. Lift your hips only as high as your weight can rest on your shoulder blades. Avoid placing weight on your neck or head.

BIRD DOG

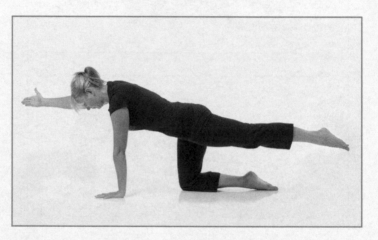

Get down on your hands and knees. Place each knee beneath each hip and each hand beneath each shoulder so that the four limbs are aligned with the four joints. Simultaneously lift your right arm and left leg, so that your leg, torso, and arm make one long diagonal line. Turn your arm inward so your palm faces your head, and turn the lifted leg inward so that the inseam of your pants moves toward the ceiling. Don't collapse into the supporting arm and leg and allow the abdomen to sag toward the floor. Instead, move your abdominals back toward your spine and puff out your lower back. Hold for five breaths, inhaling and exhaling, then switch sides. Repeat 3 to 5 times.

Benefits: Develops core strength, balance, and shoulder and hip mobility.

Caution: Lift your legs no higher than your spine. Maintain an abdominal contraction throughout to prevent "spine sag" toward the floor.

DAILY BEAT 33

BALANCE YOUR HORMONES

Throughout the last few weeks, I have talked about the fact that things like eating junk food, overexercising, and eating too quickly can all make you feel Spent. And I have mentioned that hormone balance—more accurately, hormone imbalance—is why. But now I want to talk about your hormones in a bit more depth because I believe their health and function are the pathways to either good health or feeling Spent.

Hormones are chemicals that regulate cell and organ activity. In other words, hormones are the body's heads of state—they rule how we feel and function. Most hormones are produced by various glands or organs, secreted into the bloodstream, and transported to sites where they produce a specific effect. For example, insulin is a hormone made and secreted by the pancreas. It tells cells all over the body when to use glucose (sugar) for energy. But what you might not realize is that many cells make hormones too: nerve cells, intestinal cells, heart cells, even fat cells make hormones. All of these hormones work in concert to regulate your metabolism, the rate at which your body engine runs.

Metabolism is essentially a measurement of the amount of chemical changes that take place within your body's cells, where some substances are broken down to yield energy for vital processes while other substances necessary for life are created. These chemical changes produce energy and the basic materials needed for the maintenance of all your important life processes. And as you know, when you are Spent, your metabolism is slow. It doesn't provide you with the overall energy you need to enjoy your life.

Most physicians do not consider that there is a relationship between a slowing metabolism and subtle hormonal imbalances, which are rarely diagnosed by Western medicine. More often than not, doctors relate the two only when they diagnose an overt hormonal disease such as diabetes (insulin deficiency) or Addison's disease (cortisol deficiency), which are at one extreme end of the scale. The problem with this thinking is that hormonal problems don't happen overnight. For example, it takes years before a subtle insulin imbalance (now known as metabolic syndrome or insulin resistance) becomes clinical diabetes. What's more, an insulin imbalance begins silently, without symptoms—and blood tests don't reveal this early problem. This explains why the standard blood tests for hormone levels, our only way of assessing hormone problems in Western medicine, are often an inaccurate yardstick. These tests don't pick up the subtle disruptions of hormone function, which are common when you are Spent and can lead to larger, more serious problems.

Two of the most common hormonal imbalances that are not picked up by traditional doctors and need to be addressed when someone is Spent are dysfunctional adrenal or thyroid glands. The thyroid gland is responsible for body temperature and regulates the metabolism of every cell in the body. The adrenal glands control how you react to physical, mental, and emotional stress. These two glands seem to need the most fine-tuning and, happily, are usually quite responsive to treatment.

The other two hormone systems that play an important role in Spent are insulin metabolism, which is addressed by cutting out sugar and processed foods, and the sex hormones estrogen, progesterone, and testosterone, which are often addressed automatically when we balance the adrenals and thyroid. But of course, these hormone systems are not independent. They are connected, and when one hormone is out of rhythm, the other hormones are also affected.

The most common state of hormone imbalance in Spent is one where the body is constantly trying to recover from a high-sugar, high-gluten, caffeinated diet, as well as a stressful life. When your insulin levels are bouncing up and down because you're snacking on sugary carbs, or when you live a typically stressed twenty-first-century lifestyle—particularly one in which you juggle a hectic career and family demands—your adrenal glands need to pump out cortisol and adrenaline to compensate. This perpetual state of readiness eventually exhausts your adrenals, which are working hard to deal with this constant low-grade stress. Without properly functioning adrenals, your body then loses its ability to settle down, to chill out, which stresses you out even more. So your body pumps more cortisol. This abundance of cortisol secretion then forces your thyroid to overcompensate until it reaches a point where it, too, becomes "tired" and performs sluggishly. Then you have a slower metabolism and you put on weight or find it hard to lose weight in spite of eating well and exercising. This sluggish thyroid, which helps us metabolize and digest food, then causes digestive problems, which in turn aggravate the hormonal imbalance even more! Layer onto this scenario the fact that hormone levels slowly decrease as you age, and you ultimately end up feeling as if someone has driven over you.

This story—stress, sugar, caffeine, and gluten, which are in most Americans' diets—is why I assume that hormone imbalance plays a role in nearly every patient who is Spent. This is also why I know that most of these subtle hormonal imbalances can be fixed, because they are so diet-related. After a few weeks without sugar, caffeine, gluten, processed foods, and dairy products—and with the adaptogenic formula—your body's metabolism and hormonal function are well on their way to recovery.

It is great that you are not eating sugar and gluten and drinking caffeine—and that you are doing this paired with better sleeping habits, restorative exercise, and adding a multivitamin, probiotics, the adaptogens, and fish oil. All these things will help you rebalance your hormonal system and speed up your metabolism. However, there's no one magic bullet or combination that works for everyone. There are just too many different variables that affect hormone balance because everyone is different. This is why, when searching for a patient's optimal balance, I don't stop with diet, exercise, and sleep. Instead, I continue to work toward taking as many hormone stressors as possible out of a person's life and body, lessening the total load.

The next area I address, and have already begun to address with you, is the patients' environment—from their home to their work environs. I've already asked you to think about and take some actions to detoxify your water and home, which has probably helped. But the more steps you take to purify the air, floors, and walls around you, the better you will feel. I cannot overstate the effect of the environmental pollution to which we're exposed every day. It is truly astounding and can be devastating on a hormonal level.

Synthetic chemicals build up in our bodies over the years and affect our hormonal systems in subtle and not-so-subtle ways. These chemicals disrupt our genetically programmed hormones. Remember my earlier points: our genes are designed for pure, natural foods and a certain cosmic rhythmic balance. Similarly, our genes are not used to the foreign molecules that continually assault us through the air we breathe, the personal-care and cleaning products with which we douse ourselves and our homes, and the chemicals in the food we eat and the water we drink. These foreign molecules subtly impact our hormones and, I am certain, play a formidable role in creating Spent.

I continue to urge you to make more positive changes around your home. It really is time for you to stop poisoning yourself and your hormones. We need to be living in a way that is supporting our hormonal health so that we live long, healthy, enjoyable lives. And remember, because these chemicals disrupt your metabolism, they can lead to weight gain. Women, in particular, lose weight when they start ridding their bodies of household and dietary toxins.

If you want to learn more about endocrine disruption or any of the other hormonal imbalances, go to www.spentmd.com.

The Pulse
○ • • ○ • • ○ • • ○

- Gain awareness. Begin to look around you, observing just how many toxins you come into contact with on a daily basis. Were your clothes dry-cleaned? Does your toothpaste contain fluoride? Do you use municipal water? Do you clean your kitchen counter with an environmentally safe product? What kind of toxic cleaning products does your office use? How is the air quality in your home? Do you have wall-to-wall carpeting? Are you living in a new home built with plywood and particle board that release formaldehyde, which is a toxic gas? Return to my list on page 161 of actions to take to detoxify your home, and take two more actions.

- If you have low blood pressure, crave salt, feel dizzy or light-headed when you stand up, are fatigued, and are intolerant of the cold, it could be due to poor adrenal function. In addition to an adaptogen formula, one of the best supports for our adrenals is the herb licorice root. I recommend this to nearly all of my Spent patients who have low blood pressure. If your blood pressure is low, licorice root and salt are wonderful supports for your adrenals. In addition to the adaptogens, I suggest you have a glass of water with $\frac{1}{2}$ to 1 teaspoon of salt every morning and licorice root (*Glycyrhiza glabra*) extract (standardized to 25% [150 milligrams] glycyrrhizic acid) twice a day. **Warning: *Do not* take salt or licorice root if your blood pressure is high or high normal as it can increase your blood pressure!** Side effects to look out for if you take licorice are fluid retention and a low potassium level. For more information, go to www.spentmd.com.

○ Do 40 minutes of restorative exercise outside in the sun.

○ Continue adding probiotics to your morning smoothie.

○ Continue taking a multivitamin, an adaptogenic formula, and flaxseed or fish oil.

○ Continue to follow the Spent restorative eating program, liberating your body from sugar, artificial sweeteners, processed foods, gluten, dairy products, factory-farmed meats, soy, GMO corn, mercury-laden fish, alcohol, and caffeinated beverages.

○ Take three breathing breaks today.

SLEEP BEAT

○ Turn off your TV, cell phones, and computers by 10 p.m.

○ Keep your bedroom cool. Keep the thermostat low.

○ Darken your bedroom completely or use an eye mask.

● **Practice the Hip Bridge with Cactus Arms core-strengthening exercise (page 183).** Then try the supported Savasana. In this version, your heart and chest are even more elevated. This lifting of the chest acts directly on the emotional center, helping to elevate your mood. When our chest droops down, we feel depressed, and when we are depressed, our chest droops down. The body and the mind act as one, so when we support the back in this way and open the chest we tend to feel more emotionally buoyant.

RECLINING OPEN CHEST POSE

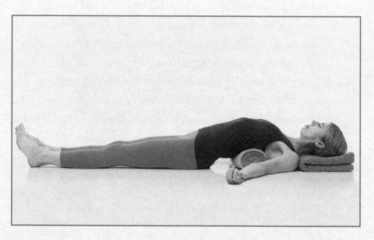

Roll up one blanket into a long, tight Tootsie Roll shape (like the one in the photograph under the model's chest). Take a second blanket and fold it in half (like the one under the model's head). Adjust the rolled blanket's position so that when you lie back, it comes to rest in the center of the upper back, just under the shoulder blades. Then lie back so that your head rests comfortably on the second folded blanket. Your head and neck should feel easy. Your throat should be relaxed and not overstretched or closed. Open and lift your chest. Stay in the pose, relaxing as in the basic Savasana, for 5 to 10 minutes. If the pose is slightly uncomfortable at first, do not worry; that will go away after a few days' practice, as tension leaves your body.

DAILY BEAT 34

REACH OUT AND TOUCH SOMEONE

In one of my first jobs as a doctor after qualifying, I was working with Paul Davis, an exceptional general practitioner in Johannesburg, South Africa. Trying to learn as much as I could, I used to follow him around in his practice. His patients adored him. I noticed early on that when he examined and talked to his patients, he would always touch them in a very reassuring way. He always used to say, "Patients get better in spite of all the drugs we give them. Your job as a physician is to be there for them and comfort them." Over the years, I've found that one of the most comforting things I can do is to touch my patients. The experience of being touched in a nonsexual way is healing. I am very lucky that I do acupuncture with my patients, where I have an appropriate reason and way to touch them. Touch is a tricky subject to talk about because our culture is so afraid of it, which is a tragedy because physical contact is so necessary for our health and well-being.

Babies don't grow properly if they are not held. Children who are not touched and hugged grow up to be more physically violent. Adults need to be touched because it builds our immune system and is emotionally soothing. The more hugs, pats on the back, and kisses on the cheek you give and receive, the better you will feel. An appropriate touch triggers the release of brain endorphins—an endogenous analgesic more powerful than heroin or morphine.

This said, I am not suggesting you make an inappropriate pass at a workmate or friend. I am talking about healing touch, where both parties feel comfortable, at ease, and even enlivened by the exchange. Old friends hugging when reuniting. Kissing someone hello or good-bye on the cheek. Snuggling with your child or partner as you read to him or her. A massage.

Some people don't like being touched, particularly on the front of the body. I completely understand some people's aversion to touch, particularly if they have been abused. And for many, the line of touch can be blurry, slipping from one intention or experience to another. So we must always be sensitive to this.

But touch is a primal human need. Many of us yearn for it. And we as a culture need to find a way back to being tender and sweet with one another so that everyone feels safe and secure and loved. Here are my suggestions for how to touch in a way that is clear and kind:

Hug friends or kiss them on the cheek. A good hug can last a week.

Walk arm in arm or hold hands with your partner, a friend, or your child.

When talking to someone, gently touch his or her arm or hand during the conversation. Such small gestures can be comforting.

Snuggle with your children, your partner, or a friend while watching television.

Give your partner a massage.

Get a massage.

A simple pat on the back can relieve a truckload of stress. Touch is a human need. And it is free.

For inspiration, check out www.freehugscampaign.org. Juan Mann (a pseudonym) walked the streets of Sydney, Australia, offering free hugs to anyone who needed one until he was banned from doing it. His free hugs campaign has become a global movement. Similarly, Ammachi, a fifty-three-year-old woman from southern India, travels the world giving hugs and is considered a living saint in her homeland. Anyone who has had a hug from her says that a hug from her is like no other. Check her out at www.ammachi.org.

The Pulse

○ • • ○ • • ○ • • ○

- Reach out and touch someone.
- Do Cross Crawl on Foam Roller, a core-strengthening exercise (page 182), before your restorative exercise.
- If you feel up to it, increase your restorative exercise practice to 45 minutes.
- If you decided to add licorice root to your daily supplement routine, begin taking it today—once in the morning and once in the afternoon.
- Try a new snack today.

SLEEP BEAT

- ○ Stay on your new sleep schedule.
- ○ Take the Spent sleep formula.
- **Go to sleep and try to wake up tomorrow morning without an alarm clock.** It can be very stressful to your body to be woken up by an alarm clock. By now your body rhythms should be better and you have been regulating your sleep so that you probably are already waking up at about the same time every day. So try not using an alarm clock and see if you really still need it. If you are stressed by the idea that you will not wake up in time to get to work, lower the volume of the alarm clock and move it across the room so that the volume and impact of the sound are decreased.
- ○ Before bed, do the Occipital Release for your neck and head (page 142). When the neck is free, it liberates the body. If you feel like adding more, do the Ultimate Neck and Shoulder Release (page 57).

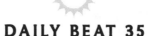

DAILY BEAT 35

FORGIVE

Archbishop Desmond Tutu says, "When I talk of forgiveness, I mean the belief that you can come out the other side a better person. A better person than the one being consumed by anger and hatred. Remaining in that state locks you in a state of victimhood, making you almost dependent on the perpetrator. If you can find it in yourself to forgive, then you are no longer chained to the perpetrator. You can move on, and you can even help the perpetrator to become a better person too." [1]

Nelson Mandela, a hero of mine and one of the truly remarkable people of our time, embodied the forgiveness that Archbishop Tutu describes. When he was released after decades of imprisonment in South Africa for the crime of wanting freedom for his people, he walked past his prison guards a free man and his first reaction was rage. How could he silently pass by the men who'd kept him a prisoner and who'd often treated him brutally? But Mandela realized that he'd already been imprisoned for nearly thirty years and that his fury at the guards would only delay his true freedom. Instead of allowing his anger to imprison him, he forgave his guards and walked into his new life as a truly free man. Later, when Mandela was inaugurated as president of the new, apartheid-free South Africa, he invited two of his prison guards to sit with him on the dais.

What both Archbishop Tutu and Nelson Mandela understand is that our resentments are more poisonous to us than to the person whom we are resenting. When we are resentful, *we* carry the rage, the upset, the hurt. And where else are we going to hold all this toxic emotion but in our bodies? If we have a big enough resentment or a list of smaller ones, how is it going to make us feel? More than likely, Spent.

Earlier on in the program, I talked about the idea that our fascia and muscles are where we hold our emotional tension and unhappiness. Although release techniques are wonderful tools, a true release is not going to happen until we let go on all levels. To experience real freedom—

physically, mentally, and emotionally—we have to make the choice to stop resenting. Not to hold on to past grudges, uncomfortable conversations, upsetting events. To move on and live in the present moment.

Of course, this is often easier said than done. For some of us, letting go of this kind of heartache means first doing some inner personal work—alone or with a therapist or even a friend—so that we can really understand and have perspective on the situation before we let it go. For others and for smaller situations, letting go of past trespasses is simply about being willing to see others as human beings—beautiful, flawed humans who are probably trying just as hard as you to move through life. You don't have to excuse their behavior, just understand that the person was possibly operating with insufficient skills. In the case of Mandela, the guards might have known that their behavior was abominable but for whatever reason were too limited to act humanely—maybe because in a system like apartheid no one feels human.

Mandela's story is a powerful reminder for me that forgiveness is the doorway to freedom. Only I can liberate myself. Only you can liberate yourself. It is a choice.

One final thought: the person we often have the hardest time forgiving is ourself. If there is something you have said or done or not said or not done, take whatever action you can to repair the problem and then forgive yourself. Let it go. To err is human. This adage holds true for you too.

The Pulse

○ ♦ ♦ ○ ♦ ♦ ○ ♦ ♦ ○

- Forgive yourself for being a wonderful and flawed human being.
- Before work, maybe try the three chair-fighting technologies (pages 157–58). The more we learn to let go with our hips, the more we can let go with our hearts.
- Do 45 minutes of restorative exercise. Listen to your body. Be mindful of your energy level.
- If you decided to include licorice root and salt to support your adrenals, continue taking them.

○ Continue taking flaxseed or fish oil.
○ Find something to laugh about or someone to laugh with today.

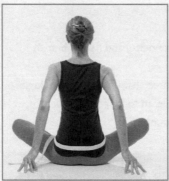

SLEEP BEAT

● Don't use an alarm clock.
● **Practice Supta Baddha Konasana with a Belt and Bolster for 10 minutes.** If I had to choose one restorative yoga pose to recommend to my patients, this would be it. It is powerfully healing because of its deep relaxing effect. It takes a bit of setting up, but anyone who has practiced this pose correctly for ten minutes will tell you that there is nothing like it. Personally, I love it; it is my all-time favorite pose when my body is tired and my mind is racing. There is something about this pose that facilitates deep relaxation.

SUPTA BADDHA KONASANA
WITH A BELT AND BOLSTER

If you have practiced the Modified Supta Baddha Konasana a couple of times, this will come easily. Study the photographs to see how the belt supports the legs. It loops around the back of your hips—not your waist—across your sacrum (see the photograph at left for the exact position) and then in between your knees and then around the outer edges of your feet.

The soles of your feet are pressed together, and the belt can be tightened

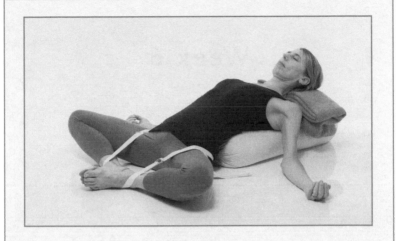

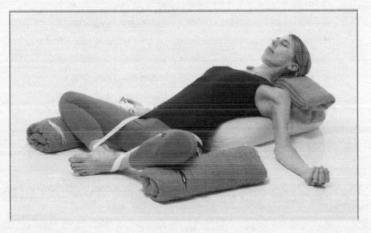

to pull the heels closer to your groin (see second photograph). Use rolled blankets, cushions, or pillows under your legs so there is no strain on your hips and your legs are fully supported (see third photograph). Set up the belt around your feet in this way and have your legs supported before you lean back centrally onto the bolster. Make sure that a folded blanket or pillow supports your head properly, as in the photographs.

Benefits: This pose is excellent for stress and exhaustion and the best pose for menstrual discomfort and indigestion.

Week 6

Sustain

A human being is part of the whole called by us universe, a part limited in time and space. We experience ourselves, our thoughts and feelings as something separate from the rest. A kind of optical delusion of consciousness. This delusion is a kind of prison for us, restricting us to our personal desires and to affection for a few persons nearest to us. Our task must be to free ourselves from the prison by widening our circle of compassion to embrace all living creatures and the whole of nature in its beauty.

—Albert Einstein

Now that you are feeling better, thanks to a more reasonable exercise program, proper diet and supplementation, and release exercises, it is time to look at ways to sustain this good feeling so that when you end the program at the end of the week, you don't crash back toward your old tired self. As my patients get better, we look at ways for them to reduce their total load so that their body's burden stays light. We get rid of more environmental toxins and make sure their cellular function is optimized and they have a healthy relationship with their bodies and work. And I will introduce the concept of Ubuntu, something near and dear to my heart.

In many ways, this is my favorite phase of work with my patients because I see their bodies and lives begin to flower.

DAILY BEAT 36

CLEAN OUT YOUR MEDICINE CABINET

We have looked at what you are putting *into* and *around* your body; now we will address what you are putting *onto* your body, because up to 60 percent of what you put on your skin can end up in your bloodstream. Between the shampoo, toothpaste, face cream, and body cream you use on a daily basis, you are combining scores of chemicals and adding to your toxic load. With regular long-term use, it is the cumulative effect that causes concern.

I know, you are attached to your products. Maybe you are even convinced that a certain cream makes you look five years younger. I'm sorry to have to be the one to tell you that, while it may be making a temporary difference, it is more than likely filled with toxic chemicals that promote disease and will ultimately accelerate your aging process. I know this all sounds a bit scary, but I'd rather you know it now rather than discover it the hard and irreversible way later. The Europeans are taking this seriously, and in 2005, a directive passed by the European Union mandated that chemicals determined to be carcinogens, mutagens, or reproductive toxins be removed from cosmetics sold in Europe.[1]

According to the Environmental Working Group, the average American is exposed to more than a hundred different chemicals from personal care products every day.[2] And although the cosmetic industry asserts that its products are safe, 89 percent of the ingredients used in cosmetics today have not been assessed by either the FDA or the industry itself.[3] This is because there are major gaps in public health laws that allow cosmetics companies to use almost any ingredient they choose with no restrictions and no requirement for safety testing.[4] Luckily for us, the Environmental Working Group researchers have created a remarkable database that pairs the ingredients in nearly 25,000 products against 50 toxicity and regulatory databases. It is a safety guide for cosmetics and personal care products. Go to www.cosmeticdatabase.com and check the cosmetics you use. Some of the ingredients in cosmetics listed in the "Not to Buy" section include lead, mercury, petroleum by-products, fragrance, nanoparticles, extracts from human and cow placenta, and phthalates.

To give you a sense of how toxic these products are, let's take a look at just a few of the most popular chemicals used in hair and skin care.

PHTHALATES AND PARABENS

Banned by the European Union in 2003, phthalates and parabens are a group of chemicals commonly used as preservatives in cosmetics. Laboratory tests found phthalates in more than 70 percent of the health and beauty products tested—including the most popular brands of hair and skin care products and every single fragrance tested. Both have been demonstrated to be carcinogenic and particularly linked to breast cancer.[5,6,7,8]

FRAGRANCE

"Fragrance" is a euphemism for nearly 4,000 different ingredients. Most "fragrances" are synthetic and are either cancer-causing or otherwise toxic. Exposure to fragrances has been shown to affect the central nervous system. "Fragrances" are found in most shampoos, deodorants, sunscreens, skin care, and body care products.

DIETHANOLAMINE (DEA) AND TRIETHANOLAMINE (TEA)

DEA and its variants are suspected of increasing the risk of cancer. DEA and TEA can combine with amines present in cosmetic formulations to form nitrosamines (N-nitrosodiethanolamine), which are known to be highly carcinogenic.[9] DEA can also show up as a contaminant in products containing related chemicals, such as cocamide DEA.

SODIUM LAURYL SULFATE (SLS) AND SODIUM LAURETH SULFATE (SLES)

Although advertised as natural and safe, I recommend you try to avoid sodium lauryl sulfate and sodium laureth sulfate, especially when used in combination with other chemicals (which they usually are). For example, when used in combination with DEA and TEA, they can form nitrosamines, which, as I said above, are a deadly carcinogen. SLS and SLES are some of the most popular ingredients in makeup, shampoo, conditioner, and toothpaste. And because they readily dissolve grease, they are also used to clean engines and garage floors and at car washes. SLS and SLES have been found to contain 1,4-dioxane, a known carcinogen.[10, 11] Though the U.S. Food and Drug Administration encourages manufacturers not to use this contaminant, it is not banned by federal law.

DIAZOLIDINYL UREA, IMIDAZOLIDINYL UREA, AND QUATERNIUM-15

These all release formaldehyde, which is what scientists and morticians use to preserve corpses and body parts. Remember dissecting frogs in school? These chemicals are linked to allergies, chest pain, chronic fatigue, depression, dizziness, ear infections, headaches, joint pain, and loss of sleep and can trigger asthma.[12, 13] They can weaken the immune system and cause cancer.[14] Diazolidinyl urea and imidazolidinyl urea are used in many skin care and hair care products. Quarternium-15 is used as a preservative in many skin and hair care products.

PETROLATUM AND MINERAL OIL (LIQUID PETROLATUM)

Petrolatum is mineral oil jelly. Mineral oil is a by-product of the distillation of petroleum to produce gasoline. This means it is a petrochemical that will coat your skin like Saran Wrap. The skin then cannot breathe, absorb, or excrete. It also slows the skin's natural cell development, causing the skin to age prematurely. Mineral oil with added "fragrance" is marketed as baby oil in the United States, United Kingdom, and Canada and is 100 percent bad for your baby's sensitive skin.

TALC

Talc is related to asbestos, a known carcinogen, and is the main ingredient in baby powder, medicated and perfumed powders, and designer perfumed body powders. Numerous studies have shown a strong link between frequent use of talc in the female genital area and ovarian cancer.[15] A National Toxicology Program study found that cosmetic-grade talc caused tumors in animal subjects.[16]

PROPYLENE GLYCOL (PG)

Propylene glycol is the active ingredient in antifreeze. It is also used in makeup, toothpaste, and deodorant. Stick deodorants have a higher concentration of PG than is allowed for most industrial use! Direct contact can cause brain, liver, and kidney abnormalities. The EPA requires workers to wear protective gloves, clothing, and goggles when working with it. Yet the FDA says we can put it into our mouths even though it has determined that it is not safe to use in or on cat food![17]

TRICLOSAN

This is a synthetic antibacterial ingredient that has been compared to Agent Orange. The Environmental Protection Agency registers it as a pesticide, highly toxic to any living organism. It is also classified as a chlorophenol. In other words, it is in a cancer-causing chemical class.[18] Triclosan disrupts hormones, can affect sexual function and fertility, and may foster birth defects.[19] It is widely used in antibacterial cleansers, toothpaste, and household products. A number of studies have found that washing with regular soap and warm water is just as effective at killing germs.[20]

NANOPARTICLES

Nanoparticles are tiny chemicals that are increasingly being used by cosmetic manufacturers as penetration enhancers because nanoparticles easily pass through the body's membranes and can reach all parts of our body. Unfortunately this also means that they may accumulate or override our normal control systems that manage our complex biochemistry, with unidentified health effects. Increasing numbers of scientific papers are demonstrating the general risks associated with nanotoxicity, yet there has been little effort on the part of regulators to slow the expansion of the nanocosmetics sector. In an extensive report dated May 2006, Friends of the Earth strongly recommends a moratorium on the further release of sunscreens, cosmetics, and personal care products containing engineered nanomaterials and the withdrawal of such products currently on the market until adequate safety studies have been completed and adequate regulations have been put in place to protect the general public.

Are you scared yet? I must admit that researching this and revisiting these facts scared me all over again. And if this were not enough, we must remember that our skin has a large surface area and is extremely permeable. So these toxins enter easily, traveling right to our bloodstream. And we keep our skin care products on for a long time—all day—so there is a greater chance of absorbing these chemicals. I believe this adds a huge burden to your health. I have seen many women who felt significantly better when they switched their skin care products. I really hope this inspires you to take on tonight's assignment: detox your medicine cabinet, looking for any and all of these chemicals. It is time to stop pouring toxins onto your head, face, and body, into your mouth (in toothpaste), and into your bloodstream.

Please note: as I said earlier, unbelievable as it may sound, here in the United States, the FDA doesn't require cosmetics companies to test their products for safety.

A final thought before I give you today's assignment:

I am a big believer in the Precautionary Principle, which is a new way of thinking and making decisions about health and the environment. Precaution comes from a Latin word meaning "to be on one's guard." The

Precautionary Principle focuses on making conscientious environmental decisions today that will have a positive effect on tomorrow—for ourselves and for our children. Why wouldn't we live this way?

The Pulse

○ • • ○ • • ○ • • ○

- Go to a health food store or a Whole Foods Market, or see the Resources section (page 305) or my Web site, www .spentmd.com, for clean cosmetics. **Buy skin and hair care products that actually care for your skin and hair.** If you are looking for a fragrance, essential oils are a wonderful alternative. Look for aluminum-free deodorant. As with everything else on this program, finding new products and your rhythm with them may take time. You may have to try one or two shampoos before you find one that works for you.

○ Do 45 minutes of restorative exercise, preferably outside.

○ Practice one core-strengthening exercise today (pages 182–84).

○ If you decided to include licorice root and salt in your program, continue taking them.

- **Continue adding probiotics to this week's Smoothie of the Week: the Cherry Peach Avocado Smoothie (page 271).**

○ Continue taking a multivitamin, an adaptogenic formula, and flaxseed or fish oil.

○ Continue to follow the Spent restorative eating program, liberating your body from sugar, artificial sweeteners, processed foods, gluten, dairy products, factory-farmed meats, soy, GMO corn, mercury-laden fish, alcohol, and caffeinated beverages.

- **Clean out your medicine cabinet.** Pitch anything containing the chemicals I discussed. If you can't bear to get rid of a certain product, finish it and then try to find a healthier replacement.

SLEEP BEAT

○ Continue not to use an alarm clock.

● Restore yourself. Today's task has the potential of being over-
stimulating and exhausting. To restore yourself and soothe
your nervous system, practice the second version of Viparita
Karani. This is one of the most refreshing and soothing restorative yoga poses I know. There is nothing like it after a hard
day's work or when your legs are tired.

VIPARITA KARANI II

*Skill is needed to get into this pose. If you don't get it right the first time, with
your buttocks touching or very close to the wall, do not be surprised. It takes a
few tries.*

*Set the bolster three to five inches from the wall, depending on how flex-
ible you are. As in the first picture in the sequence on the following pages, sit
on one end of the bolster with your hip touching the wall. Then lie down on
your side, roll onto your back with bent knees, and extend your legs up the
wall. If your head is on a hard surface, you may want to place a folded blanket
or towel under it. If you do do this, be sure that your chin is parallel with the
floor. Stay in the pose for 5 to 10 minutes.*

Note: *This can also be practiced with one or two blankets folded to make
the same long rectangular shape as a bolster.*

Caution: *Do not practice this pose during menstruation.*

(continued on next page)

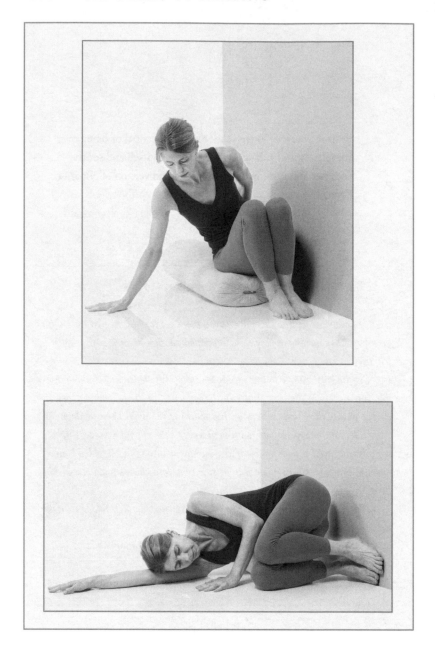

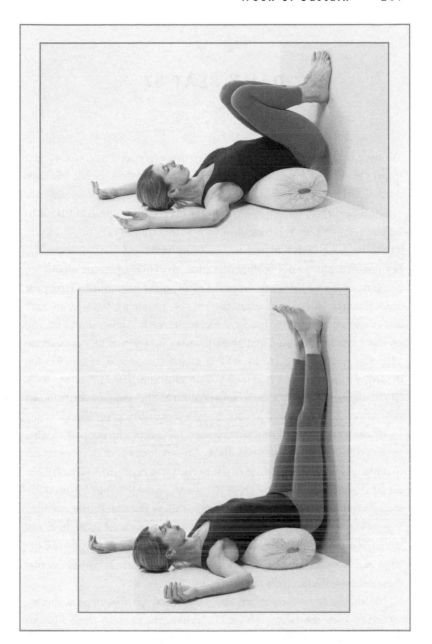

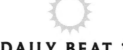

DAILY BEAT 37

GO CELLULAR

We have been working hard—and on nearly every level—to restore you to your sparkling former self. As you may have noticed, in the last few days, my suggestions have become about the more subtle and refined ways we can heal Spent and restore rhythm. Today is even more specific. I want to look at cell function. You have about a hundred trillion cells in your body. These are your body's most basic building blocks. If your cells are not healthy, then you are not healthy, and, more than likely, you are Spent.

One of the best ways to support healthy cell function is to feed your mitochondria. Mitochondria are the energy-producing factories in each and every cell. They assimilate food molecules, such as glucose and fat, and produce crucial nutrients. But their primary function is to manufacture adenosine triphosphate (ATP). ATP is a vital component of life. Among the many roles it plays, it facilitates cell division and synthesizes our DNA. Essentially, ATP functions as the universal form of chemical energy in our cells, which fuels every cell in your body—sort of like a "life force."

Picture each cell as a tiny factory assembly line producing part of what we call our life. Each of these assembly lines requires continuous supplies of raw materials for its productivity. If needed raw materials aren't available for a particular assembly line, these items are usually scavenged from other areas. In the worst-case scenario, the output stops. But usually the assembly line will take whatever bits and pieces it can get, which are sometimes not the right supplies. When this happens, the end product is obviously not the same and fatigue is usually one of the results. Therefore it is essential that these cells receive the right raw materials.

As in any factory, there are also waste products that need to be removed to keep the factory clean. The cell works to clean these from its environment so that the body can eliminate them. If a cell does not do all it is supposed to do to keep the factory clean, it will begin to function less optimally and fatigue will result.

To keep the factory functioning optimally and prevent "cellular fatigue," we need to give the cells the nutrients they need, ensure that they are getting rid of waste products, and see that they are communicating well with other parts of the assembly line (the other cells).

Optimal mitochondrial energy production prevents cellular fatigue and is essential for physical strength, energy, stamina, and life itself. Even the slightest drop in mitochondrial energy output, no matter how subtle, can lead to weakness, fatigue, and cognitive difficulties. Unfortunately, when you're under stress and as you age, mitochondrial function—like just about everything else—becomes less efficient. Interestingly, exercise improves mitochondrial function.

If you are still tired after five weeks on this program, it may be because you have cellular fatigue and your mitochondria may need more of a boost. Fortunately, in addition to exercise, there is an easy supplement solution for this. Researchers have found that a few key nutrients can improve mitochondrial function.[21, 22, 23] These include coenzyme Q10, alpha-lipoic acid, acetyl-L-carnitine, and some of the B vitamins. Fish oils are also essential because when we don't have enough omega-3 fatty acids, our cell walls take up the wrong type of fat, which affects cellular function and leads to cellular fatigue. You should already be taking B vitamins in your multivitamin and getting extra omega-3s in flaxseed or fish oil supplements.

Here are some more supplements that can improve your mitochondrial function.

COENZYME Q10 (COQ10)

Also known as "ubiquinone," CoQ10 is essential for the production of energy in every cell of your body. It also helps your body maintain higher levels of vitamin C and E. CoQ10 is found naturally in beef, soy, sardines, mackerel, peanuts, and organ meats. I recommend 100 to 200 milligrams of CoQ10 a day. (It's especially important if you're also taking a statin drug to lower cholesterol, because these drugs can deplete CoQ10 levels.)

ALPHA-LIPOIC ACID (ALA)

Like CoQ10, ALA is a nutrient produced naturally by the body; its production also decreases as we age. It helps cells metabolize energy and acts as a powerful antioxidant. What's more, ALA "recycles" other key antioxidants, such as vitamin C, vitamin E, and glutathione. Red meat and organ meats (heart and liver) are the richest dietary sources of alpha-lipoic acid, but it is also present in small amounts in potatoes, carrots, yams, beets, and spinach. I recommend 200 to 400 milligrams a day.

CARNITINE AND ACETYL-L-CARNITINE

As with CoQ10 and ALA, you need much more carnitine as you age, especially after age forty. Carnitine functions as a building block for your cells' energy-producing engine, contributing to the process that converts fatty acids into energy. Beef is the best source of carnitine, so vegetarians are especially likely to have a carnitine deficiency. Classic symptoms of carnitine deficiency include reduced ability to exercise and rapid onset of fatigue, weakness, and muscle pain after exercise. When I hear that, a good dose of carnitine usually does the trick. I recommend 1 to 3 grams of carnitine or 500 to 1,500 milligrams a day of acetyl-L-carnitine. Start at the lower dose and increase until you feel a difference. Don't take it after lunchtime because of its energizing effects; it may cause insomnia.

Together, acetyl-L-carnitine and alpha-lipoic acid have been found to rejuvenate mitochondrial function almost to youthful levels.[24] More good news: taking carnitine and fish oils often helps you lose weight.

If you are still feeling Spent, you may want to add coenzyme Q10, alpha-lipoic acid, or carnitine. All three are expensive but are helpful at the correct doses. Don't take suboptimal doses, as they won't be effective. You may find ALA and carnitine together in a supplement.

The Pulse

○ ● ● ○ ● ● ○ ● ● ○

- Do the Cats and Dogs stretch (page 143) to wake your body up.
- ○ Do 45 minutes of restorative exercise today.
- ○ Practice one core-strengthening exercise today (pages 182–84) to support your posture.
- If you decided to add coenzyme Q10, alpha-lipoic acid, and/or acetyl-L-carnitine to support and heal mitochondrial function, go to your local health food store and buy one or two of them. Or go to www.spentmd.com for my favorites.
- ○ Continue taking a multivitamin, an adaptogenic formula, and flaxseed or fish oil.
- If you feel you need it, take an hour of quiet time for yourself today to do whatever you want: listen to music, meditate, read.

SLEEP BEAT

- ○ Continue not using an alarm.
- Practice the Spinal Reset (page 81) and do the Side-Lying Spine Rotation with Arm Circles (page 108) before bed, or, while lying on the foam roller in the Spinal Reset, include some arm circles. This way you will get more of a release.

DAILY BEAT 38

SLOW DOWN

A week or so ago, I talked about using music to chill out and to illustrate the fact that the body and mind can actually be slowed down by the steady beats of music. This mechanism to mimic or unite with a pulse greater than our own is called "entrainment."

Try counting your heart rate or breathing rate when you're in traffic, around noisy machinery, or listening to loud rock music. Then count your heart rate or breathing rate when you are sitting quietly on a beach or listening to peaceful music in a peaceful surrounding. Our internal rhythms speed up or slow down to match the stronger external rhythm around us. In fact, the external rhythms and our bodies' inner rhythms or pulses are inseparable.

We are entraining to our surroundings and the rhythms around us all the time but are not aware of it; it's not a conscious thing. It is part of our lives, so subtle that we take it for granted and don't notice it. However, you may notice it when you travel—it takes a few days to find the pace of the beach, city, or country you are in. Beyond recovering from jet lag, it is your body entraining to the local rhythm. For instance, whenever I go away, especially to the beach, it takes me a few days to get into the rhythm of the location. Usually about the third day, I notice I am walking more slowly, moving more slowly, talking more slowly, and generally being slower than I am in New York. I become entrained to the slowly lapping water and easier pace.

Throughout the last few weeks, I have talked about the various ways in which you were entrained to the fast-paced rhythm of modern life and the fact that your genes are not programmed to function at such a fast pace. I have worked on nearly every level to get you to slow down. I have wanted you to begin to entrain your body back to a slower rhythm that has more to do with nature than with concrete sidewalks and racing traffic. By immersing yourself in a better environment—with meditation, spending more time outside in the sun, breathing breaks, getting more sleep, eating more consciously—your body has, hopefully, been restored to a more even, slower, steadier rhythm and, as a result, is feeling better. There is a reason why you have more energy.

In physics less energy is used when two objects are entrained with each other. In other words, we expend less energy when we are in step with the surrounding energy. Yes, we might need to speed up if we need to at work or if the energy of work is fast, but we also need to be able to slow down when we come home. As with restorative exercise, but on a larger scale, we need to teach the body to slow down, to relax, to recover, to stimulate the parasympathetic system. We need to find external rhythms that are slow (nature, quiet surroundings, certain music) that we can entrain to as well, because when we are Spent, we tend to live in overdrive.

Like consuming sugar or caffeine, being busy is a vice. I have seen how being busy keeps me and many of my patients from knowing or being alone with their feelings. Being reflective or contemplative has somehow become scary. My experience has been that most people deny or are not aware that their busyness is a way of distracting themselves from issues in their lives. Instead, they exercise, eat, drink, go online, or do things such as gamble to distract themselves. Unfortunately, this desire to remain unaware and out of touch with who we really are ultimately fails and we become emotionally Spent. To heal, we are forced to look at whatever it is that we are avoiding.

In a conversation with the philosopher and Nobel Laureate Bertrand Russell, the Dalai Lama said, "Let us reflect on what is truly of value in life, what gives meaning to our lives, and set our priorities on the basis of that. The purpose of our life needs to be positive. We weren't born with the purpose of causing trouble, harming others. For our life to be of value, I think we must develop basic good human qualities—warmth, kindness, compassion. Then our life becomes meaningful and more peaceful—happier."

Slowing down allows us to listen for and find our real values and goals so that we can realize our most authentic selves.

The Pulse

○ ● ● ○ ● ● ○ ● ● ○

- **Allow yourself to slow down.** Wait a few rings before you answer the phone, take a few breaths or just sit quietly for a moment before lunch, sit in your car for a few minutes and breathe or listen to music before going home from work. Whatever job you have to do, slow down and do it well. I think you'll actually notice that if you don't rush, things will get done more easily because the body doesn't also need to manage frenetic energy as it accomplishes task after task.
- **To help you really slow down, practice the One Global Breath Meditation for 10 minutes. See www.spentmd.com.**
- **Take the day off from your restorative exercise.**
- ○ Do one core-strengthening exercise today (pages 182–84).
- ○ If you decided to add coenzyme Q10, alpha-lipoic acid, and/or acetyl-L-carnitine to support and heal mitochondrial function, begin or continue taking one or more of them.
- ○ Remember to add color to your diet.

SLEEP BEAT

- **Do something to help you chill out. Meditate. Listen to your favorite music. Take a bath. Cook.**
- ○ Turn off your TV, cell phones, and computers by 10 p.m.
- ○ Keep your bedroom cool. Keep the thermostat low.
- ○ Darken your bedroom completely or use an eye mask.
- **To see how your core exercises are working, do a Posture Check on the Floor (see page 79).**

DAILY BEAT 39

MEDITATE WITH NATURE

Sometimes lying still and minding our breath is not what we need. Sometimes we need to move around and notice our surroundings. Sometimes a meditation with nature is the cure. To the cynics, this idea of meditating with nature may seem a little hokey, but I strongly suggest you try it. This nature walk has helped even the most city-minded, cynical patient of mine to overcome stress. It is about becoming more sensitive to your environment and the extraordinary fact that you are alive.

Today I want you to move and to be moved. To be engaged and engrossed in and with all that you do. To feel your relationship with all that is around you. When we realize our connection with everything around us and really let ourselves feel it, we cannot help but become overwhelmed with gratitude and joy.

The Pulse

○ • • ○ • • ○ • • ○

○ To wake up your body, do the Wall Stretch on page 72.

○ If have you decided to add coenzyme Q10, alpha-lipoic acid, and/or acetyl-L-carnitine to support mitochondrial function, begin or continue taking one or more of them.

● Practice the Meditation with Nature. Maybe make this your restorative exercise for the day.

● Today take this connection with the trees and the grass and extend it to feeling connected to the people around you. Even if you don't have time to go to a park or nearby woods, read the meditation through and then go through your day as though you were in the woods, seeing everything for the first time.

MEDITATION WITH NATURE

As with the previous meditation, read the instructions a few times through and then just let go and try. Your version and interpretation of the directions are all you need.

1. Find a park, woods, a beach, a nature preserve, or a reservoir. Note: *In a pinch, you can do this in your home or apartment. Tune in to the details of the space.*

2. Depending upon your time schedule, give yourself 15 minutes or half an hour.

3. Depending upon where you are, take your shoes off or keep them on.

4. Forget about the benefits of exercise.

5. Forget about what happened this morning or today before you read this.

6. Try not to anticipate what is going to happen next.

7. Walk around for a few minutes until you come to a place where you feel like pausing.

8. When you arrive at your location, focus on what is around you. When you find the place, stop.

9. Stand still for a moment and take in what is around you. Notice where you are. Take in everything—the trees, grass, sand, water, sounds, the texture of the air. Take 10 deep breaths, inhaling through the nose and exhaling through the mouth.

10. After a few more breaths, allow your feet to become more sensitive to what they are touching—the rocks under your shoes and socks, the sand under your feet, the grass between your toes. Feel where your weight is. Maybe it is more over your heels. Maybe you are leaning forward slightly.

11. Notice how your body feels. What feels sticky, tired, achy? What parts feel loose and easy? Take five more breaths, directing the breath to the sticky places. If your hips feel tight, inhale, picturing the breath traveling down and into the hips, then exhale, picturing the tension and pain streaming out of the hip socket. Likewise, if your shoulders feel as if they are rolled forward, inhale, bringing the breath into the shoulder

socket, and exhale, imagining the shoulders easing back into their sockets, the shoulder blades sliding down the back.

12. *With this newfound spaciousness, begin walking again.*

13. *For the remaining minutes, allow yourself to be completely absorbed by what is in front of you, beside you, under you, behind you. Look at the bark on the trees, the stones in the sand, a spiderweb, a flower's pistil, the shape of seaweed, the shape of your footprint, the length of your stride. Become sensitive to where the air is meeting your skin—maybe on your face and hands. Let yourself be curious about everything. If you wonder what is under a rock, look. If you want to know what kind of tree one is, move in closer and study it. If you wonder about an animal, stop and watch it. Listen for the wind, the birds, your breath.*

14. *When you are done, notice how you feel. Maybe your breath is easier. Maybe you are more relaxed. Maybe you feel more connected.*

SLEEP BEAT

○ Stay on your new sleep schedule.

○ Continue not using an alarm.

● Choose two of your favorite releases and practice them tonight: the Ultimate Neck and Shoulder Release (page 57), Neck and Shoulder Release Using a Foam Roller (page 125), hip releases (pages 157–58), or Ultimate Foot Massage (page 92).

DAILY BEAT 40

DETERMINE YOUR SENSITIVITY

As you near the end of the six-week program, you are, I hope, feeling much, much better and are probably looking forward to getting back to having some bread and cheese in your life, which in most cases will be no problem. But before we get there, I want to talk to you about why it is a good idea to take it slow when transitioning out of this six-week program—particularly when it comes to your diet.

Though more than likely you are not allergic to any of the foods you used to eat, you may be sensitive to or intolerant of them. In fact, your sensitivity to certain foods may have led you to become Spent. Signs of food sensitivity include:

- *Unexplained fatigue*
- *Unexplained dermatological symptoms*
- *Unexplained neurological symptoms*
- *Unexplained gastrointestinal symptoms*
- *Unexplained joint and muscle pains*
- *Unexplained urological symptoms*
- *Unexplained ear, nose, throat, and respiratory symptoms*
- *Fluid retention and daily fluctuations in weight*
- *Chronic mucus production*
- *Recurrent infections*
- *Anxiety, irritability, hyperactivity, inability to concentrate, and mood swings*

The difference between a food allergy and a food sensitivity is best explained by our reactions to the food. For instance, when we are allergic to a food, we usually have an immediate response (within two hours) whereas a food sensitivity can happen anywhere from two hours to three days later. A sensitivity to a food usually begins in adulthood, whereas allergies manifest themselves early in our childhood. Food sensitivities often cause digestive problems. Allergies, for the most part, do not. With food sensitivities, the amount of food needed to create symptoms is generally much larger than for food allergies, where a person can react to just a trace of the food. Finally, with food sensitivities, the reactions or symptoms can be different—swelling one time and a bad stomach another—whereas with allergies, the body consistently has the same reaction, even though, in different ways, both of these reactions involve the immune system.

We can have an even subtler reaction to food called an intolerance. The majority of "toxic" responses to food are caused by food intolerances rather than allergies or sensitivities. A food intolerance is defined as any reproducible, toxic response to food that does not involve the immune system. Food intolerance responses can occur for many different reasons. A food can contain a molecule that your body has difficulty breaking down or digesting. As that molecule is allowed to continue down your intestinal tract, your body shows signs of an intolerance response. Lactose intolerance is an example of this type of toxic food response. Food intolerances can also be caused by food additives such as benzoates (including sodium benzoate, an additive found in literally thousands of processed foods) and sulfites, which are added to processed foods to extend their shelf life. Processed foods can also contain small amounts of food residues that are not listed on the label and often colors and flavorings, which more than likely cause problems too. So how a food has been processed, handled, stored, and even prepared can have an effect on whether it will cause an intolerance reaction or not.

But for our purposes today, it does not matter if you are sensitive to or intolerant of certain foods, the results are the same: if we continuously eat foods we react to, we become sick and then, eventually, Spent. Many times people think they are eating a healthy diet, all organic, whole grains, which looks great on paper, but actually it is not healthy for them because they are sensitive to wheat or intolerant of soy. In other words, the foods that are healthy for me may be harmful for you. The old saying "One man's food is another man's poison" could not be more true.

Because of food sensitivity and intolerances, I will be asking you to take your time as you move out of this six-week program and into yet another new phase of eating. Rather than diving into a plate of pasta or a wheel of Brie in two days, I want you to reintroduce your foods slowly so that you can test for sensitivities and intolerances. I will talk more about how to do this in the coming week, but for now, know that you have done an extraordinary thing by eliminating sugar, processed foods, gluten, alcohol, caffeine, dairy products, factory-farmed meats and poultry, soy, GMO corn, and mercury-laden fish from your diet. By doing this, you have given your body—particularly your digestive system and hormones—an amazing and much-needed break. And because they have been resting, we want to wake them up slowly.

The Pulse
○ ● ● ○ ● ● ○ ● ● ○

- ○ Continue to follow the Spent restorative eating program, liberating your body from sugar, artificial sweeteners, processed foods, gluten, dairy products, factory-farmed meats, soy, GMO corn, mercury-laden fish, alcohol, and caffeinated beverages. You are almost there!
- ○ If you decided to add coenzyme Q10, alpha-lipoic acid, or acetyl-L-carnitine to support mitochondrial function, continue taking one or more of them.
- ○ If you decided to include licorice root and salt in your program, continue taking them.
- ○ Continue adding (or taking) probiotics with your morning smoothie.
- ○ Continue taking a multivitamin, an adaptogenic formula, and flaxseed or fish oil.
- ○ Do 45 minutes of restorative exercise outside.

SLEEP BEAT

- ● Practice your favorite restorative yoga pose for 10 to 15 minutes before bed.

DAILY BEAT 41

IT IS YOUR PRACTICE

Even though you say your practice is not good enough, there is no
other practice for you right now. Good or bad, it is your practice.
—Shunryu Suzuki, *Not Always So*

It has been four weeks since you started your restorative exercise program. How do you feel?

Years ago, when I first started yoga practice, I loved the effects, but I also hated it. My body couldn't do half the poses—my hips and shoulders were unbelievably tight, and I felt as if I had no arms and legs. But because I could not get a new body and desperately wanted the one I had to feel better, there was nowhere to go but back to class. So I kept going to classes and things got better. But my hips are still tight and my shoulders could still use some opening, and that is the way it is. That is the way it has been for me and all forms of exercise. I am not David Beckham or Roger Federer.

Most of us—especially people who love exercise or moving—want our bodies to be stronger, faster, suppler, lither, freer, more capable, and easier with whatever challenges we give them. Well, I'm sorry to be the one to tell you that satisfaction is rarely the case.

Either we can be unhappy, or we can think again and be happy with where we are with our bodies, the restorative yoga, posture exercises, and restorative exercise—whether you are jogging or walking for an hour and doing all of the restorative yoga or have just worked up to 35 minutes of brisk walking and strolling and have done the Spinal Reset only once or twice.

Unlike the diet, I have not given you strict directions for how to practice your restorative exercise, yoga, and posture work, mostly because I know that most people will either not do it or overexert themselves. I have tried to stay out of your head and away from giving you a goal. The goal for exercise is to feel better and stronger. Period. The end.

If your restorative exercise regimen is tiring you out and you tend to overdo, slow down. And if you know you are not doing enough, well, do a bit more. It's really up to you.

Will you dare to let yourself be happy with where you are? Will you dare to let yourself feel good?

The Pulse

○ • • ○ • • ○ • • ○

- **Revise your restorative exercise program so that it better suits your needs.** Maybe commit to doing an hour of walking for 4 minutes and jogging for 2. Maybe commit to walking briskly for 1 minute and strolling for 1 minute for 50 minutes. Maybe commit to adding a few more core exercises such as the Bird Dog (page 184) or releasing the shoulders more with the Ultimate Neck and Shoulder Release (page 57).
- **Take another step to detoxify your home and clean up your personal care products.**

SLEEP BEAT

○ Stay on your new sleep schedule and continue not using an alarm clock.

- **Open your heart more. Practice the Supported Savasana on page 105 for 10 to 15 minutes.** When you are in the pose, watch your breath. If negative thoughts interrupt you, practice thinking again. Aim for being with what is: the stiff back, the tight shoulders, a sore knee, your belly, your ankles. Try to engender a sense of gratitude for your body. For better or worse, it is your home.

DAILY BEAT 42

PRACTICE UBUNTU

As a doctor, especially one who spends an enormous amount of time and energy researching, talking about, and treating diseases that are a result of our unhealthy environment, I know that it is essential to my health and the health of my patients to have a positive outlook and to see the beauty in the world. There are many ways to do this—dancing, listening to music, spending time with family and friends—but I believe the mother of all of these activities is doing something useful and meaningful to you.

I am blessed to have found great meaning in my family and work, but I have found that becoming involved with organizations that are making a difference on the planet is extraordinarily satisfying and healing too. I feel empowered and connected, and with these groups I see the beauty of this very messy world.

In South Africa, there is a word, Ubuntu, which Archbishop Desmond Tutu describes as "what it means to be truly human, to know that you are bound up with others in the bundle of life, for a person is only a person through other people."

Ubuntu is humaneness, it is kindness, understanding, compassion, tolerance, caring, sharing, sensitivity, and respect all in one. It is a distinctly African social ethic, a way of relating to others. It means that what makes us human is the humanity we show one another, a worldview that sees humanity as a web of family rather than a mass of individuals. We are all related, interdependent, and connected.

I first learned about this concept when I was working as a physician in KwaNdebele, South Africa, in 1981 and 1982. During apartheid, KwaNdebele was a "homeland" where the government forced the local Ndebele tribe (and others) to live. When I drove into the rural areas to get to the various clinics where I would see patients, even though I was a white man they didn't know, I was never seen as a symbol of white oppression—amazing, given the suffering the people living there were enduring. Wherever I stopped along the way, people invited me into their homes for a meal, even if they had hardly anything. Whatever they had, they offered to share. This was a profound experience for me. They, unlike my white counterparts, saw and acknowledged our connection. My hunger was their hunger.

To this day, Ubuntu provides me with a powerful perspective: it gets the focus off myself, my suffering, my problems and reconnects me with a larger whole. It reminds me that no one can be truly healthy, wealthy, and wise if others are suffering.

I believe that participating in something you truly believe in is the final and, in some way, ultimate answer to healing Spent. This is particularly true for those who work at a high-pressure job—banking, real estate, advertising—or in a profession that doesn't feel meaningful. It is emotionally draining and, I believe, detrimental to work at a job that does not align with your passions, beliefs, and desires.

An extreme example of what happens when a person shifts from not caring about his or her work to caring is when I told a financially successful former patient who was completely Spent (she practically crawled into my office) to quit her job and go to Africa (sort of as a joke). Six months later, I got a call from her telling me she had followed my instruction, gone to Africa, fallen in love with the people, and was now working for a nonprofit organization there—and she was feeling fantastic! And she is not the only one. I have seen this kind of transformation a number of times— people giving up their high-powered jobs, switching to something more meaningful to them, and not feeling Spent anymore. Though I am not suggesting you quit your job today, I do want you to be involved with something you care about. I can't tell you how many times I have seen people find their passion, feel connected to their work and cause, and weeks—sometimes even days—later, they are miraculously better.

In many ways, finding meaning is like falling in love. You have a certain glow. You smile more. Maybe they are the same thing? I don't know. What I do know is that if you want to feel better, helping others will probably help you as much as, if not more than, whomever you are helping.

Moreover, when people learn to give or start volunteering and caring for others, they in turn learn how to really care for themselves as well.

And finally, when you start becoming more proactive about the problems in the world, they don't overwhelm you or depress you as much because you have the sense that you can make a difference.

And you already have. Just look at how getting better has helped those around you. You are in a better mood, have more energy and more time, are more centered—and this is just the beginning!

The Pulse
○ ● ● ○ ● ● ○ ● ● ○

- **Spend half an hour exploring an organization or an idea that you think you would like to become involved with.** Look on the Internet. Make a phone call. Talk to your partner or a friend. Maybe make a commitment to get involved together. Check out the Resources section (page 305) and www .spentmd.com for links to how to get involved.
○ If you decided to add coenzyme Q10, alpha-lipoic acid, or acetyl-L-carnitine to support mitochondrial function, continue taking them.
○ If you decided to include licorice root and salt to support your adrenals, continue taking them.
○ Practice your restorative exercise outside.
○ Continue adding probiotics to your morning smoothie to support your digestion.
○ Continue taking a multivitamin, an adaptogenic formula, and flaxseed or fish oil to help your body absorb and process nutrients more effectively.
○ Continue to follow the Spent restorative eating program, liberating your body from sugar, artificial sweeteners, processed foods, gluten, dairy products, factory-farmed meats, soy, GMO corn, mercury-laden fish, alcohol, and caffeinated beverages. It's just one more day before you begin reintroducing foods. You made it!

SLEEP BEAT

○ Turn off your TV, cell phones, and computers by 10 p.m. to eliminate EMF radiation and decrease brain stimulation.

○ Keep your bedroom cool. Keep the thermostat low to optimize sleep hormones.

○ Darken your bedroom completely or use an eye mask, for uninterrupted melatonin production.

○ Stay on your new sleep schedule and continue not using an alarm clock, to support your body's natural rhythms.

○ Take the Spent sleep formula to soothe your nervous system.

● **Practice the ultimate heart-opening restorative pose.** This valuable pose improves digestion and refreshes the abdominal organs. It opens the chest, helps you breathe more deeply, and increases circulation. It needs a little setup, but it is very worthwhile taking the time to learn it.

SUPPORTED BRIDGE POSE

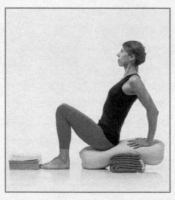

In addition to your blankets and bolster, you will need a little pile of books, about six inches high, tied with string, if you want something to rest your heels on.

This pose might need a few tries before you get it right. Look carefully at the pictures and see that you will need to place your bolster on top of a little pile of neatly folded blankets. Looking at the sequence, see how, in the first position, you need to sit centrally, quite near the end of the bolster. Keeping your knees bent at this point,

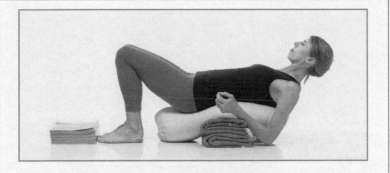

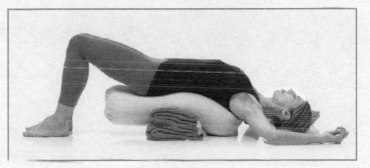

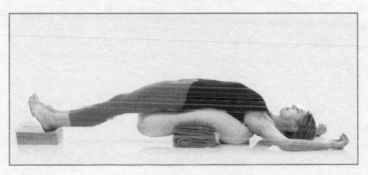

lie back so that you stay centered on the bolster and your shoulders touch the floor lightly. Then straighten your legs and place your heels on the pile of books.

Rest in the pose with your eyes closed as in the basic Savasana (see page 75) for 5 to 10 minutes. Come out of the pose by sliding off the bolster toward your head.

PART III

Staying Unspent

What to Do Now

Life is about rhythm. We vibrate, our hearts are pumping blood, we are a rhythm machine, that's what we are.

—Mickey Hart

Congratulations, you have finished the six-week restorative program for healing Spent! If you are *not* feeling vastly better, skip this chapter for now and jump right to the Troubleshooting chapter (page 241), which will work with you to root out the underlying issues that are still preventing you from feeling terrific. If you are feeling much, much better, that is great. More than likely, you are probably wondering, "What do I do now? Do I have to live like this the rest of my life to keep feeling good?" Briefly, yes and no.

As you know, the main goal of the Spent six-week program was to nudge you back to your genetically inclined, nature-driven rhythm. As I have talked about many times now, for many hundreds of generations, we were hunters and gatherers, living according to nature's daily, monthly, and seasonal cycles, living with nature's rhythms. These cycles and rhythms are imprinted in our genes and therefore in the physiology of our bodies. In other words, in our genes we are still hunters and gatherers, but we live in a world whose pace and rhythm are completely foreign to them. One of my favorite facts is that animals that live in the wild do not develop chronic diseases—in fact, neither did preindustrial humans, when they still lived in accordance to nature's rhythms—but caged animals in zoos and household pets do. It's just another sign that living in tune with our environment and genes is the key to any living being's health and wellness.

These last six weeks have been about showing you ways to become more attuned to the natural world around you—even if you live amid concrete and fluorescent lights. Among many other ideas, I have talked about the importance of day and night, eating with the seasons, our body's circadian cycle, and our breathing. Hopefully, after completing the program, you are more tuned in to the planet's rhythm and your own pulse. Maybe you even feel as if your body clock has been reset. Actually, I hope so!

I am reiterating the idea of rhythm again and reminding you of your genetic predispositions because, despite our best intentions, the tendency is to drift away from nature. Practically speaking, it is often easier to live in our modern society in a way that does not match a natural, genetically supportive rhythm. Catching up on work in front of a bright computer screen until the wee hours of the morning, misusing exercise, and eating processed foods is convenient—until we feel Spent. I say all this because your first and primary goal of what to do next is not to lose this precious rhythm that you have worked very hard to reestablish. It would be a shame for you to have done all this work and then return to the way you lived before, only to find yourself feeling Spent again in a month or so. Sure, you can now pick up some old habits, but do this cautiously, consciously (I will tell you how shortly). Maintain an awareness that you could throw yourself into the Spent zone more easily than you think, as you have only just begun to recover and reap the benefits of the program. Your newfound energy will only build.

Here are my tips for keeping and building upon this newfound rhythm. I will begin with what you should do about eating now, as this is what my patients always want to know first. Then I will continue on, answering and speaking to the greatest hits of the most frequently asked post-six-week-restorative-program questions.

What Can I Eat Now?

The next phase of eating after following the Spent restorative eating program is to begin to reintroduce foods. Here's how to do it.

Reintroduce foods in the opposite order from how you eliminated them. Reintroduce soy first, then organic corn, then dairy, then gluten. Generally speaking (birthdays and special occasions aside), it is a good idea to continue staying away from processed foods, factory-farmed meats, and sugar as much as possible.

Reintroduce soy, organic corn, dairy, and gluten over the course of two weeks or so, preferably one at a time every three days. The reason I suggest this is that if you are reactive to a food, your body is usually extra-sensitive to it after you have cleared it from your system. If you are reactive, sensitive, or allergic to a food, your reaction will be quite noticeable, even dramatic. Most reactions occur within a few hours of eating, although occasionally it can take up to two to three days for a reaction to happen. That is why I like to space out the reintroductions. This process allows you to know what food is a problem food and exhausts your body. Women should not try reintroducing foods premenstrually or during menstruation because the body is more sensitive at that time.

When testing for your sensitivity or intolerance of food, have a good serving for breakfast and lunch. That way you will know with certainty if you are reactive or not to that particular food.

Know what a food reaction looks and feels like. Common symptoms include fatigue, headache, mood changes, brain fog, sleep disturbances, digestive symptoms, puffiness, muscle and joint pains, and skin rashes. If you have a bad reaction when testing for sensitivity or intolerance, try two tablets of Alka Seltzer Gold or a tablespoon of buffered vitamin C to alleviate the symptoms. If you do have a reaction, note the symptoms and avoid that food for another three months. If when you reintroduce it after another three months, you still have symptoms, I would advise you to avoid that food altogether. If your reaction is less severe, you might want to have that food only on rare occasions.

Keep a food diary. I know, I hate this suggestion too. It is a pain. But documenting what and when you eat and what you feel and what symptoms you experience is an invaluable resource.

Even if after reintroducing these foods that we eliminated on the Spent restorative eating program, you feel fine, I still don't recommend eating soy, dairy products, or gluten more often than once every three or four days.

In terms of drinking alcohol after this program, wait until you have reintroduced the other foods, and then you can add a bit of alcohol to your diet. But I would suggest only one or two drinks a week; a maximum of three is my recommendation. More than this will disturb your body rhythms. Also, remember that beer contains gluten and wine contains sulfites. If you have discovered that you are sensitive or reactive to gluten, it is best to avoid beer.

As for caffeine, it has no nutritional value. In fact, it depletes your energy over time because it stimulates your stress hormones and also messes with your rhythms. Other than an occasional cappuccino or latte (if you are not dairy-sensitive), I don't recommend bringing it back into your life. My attitude toward caffeine is that if you don't need it, then drinking coffee now and then is no problem. If you need a cup of coffee to get you going in the morning, know that it is a sign that you are out of balance. Stop the coffee, have a cup of tea (the caffeine is not as considerable), and consider how you need to nourish your body so that you don't need this kind of boost. More sleep? More protein and healthy fats? Exercise?

Guidelines for Spent-free Eating and Living

Once you have reintroduced soy, organic corn, dairy, gluten, and a bit of alcohol, you can begin the process of refining your rhythm for the long term. Just to remind you, your body's needs during the day and night are completely different. During the day, we want the nutrients to keep us energized and alert. Protein and the amino acids into which protein breaks down are essential for this. At night, the body's main functions are to repair, restore, heal, maintain, and detox. For this, the body needs carbohydrates to help sustain your sugar levels and help you sleep. Interestingly, carbohydrates also help with the absorption of tryptophan and other nutrients that are needed for sleep.[1] So all of this means that you should eat:

- *Protein and fat in the morning. These are essential for energy. If you feel you really want a grain or a cereal for breakfast, have it only as a side dish. Having a large breakfast of appropriate foods is healthy. Remember, the first meal sets the day's rhythm. As you know, I think a smoothie is the perfect breakfast food. It contains fat and pro-*

tein and is full of phytonutrients. Note: Most commercial smoothies are nutritionally empty and loaded with sugar, which is why I have given you so many options in the back of the book.

- A mixed greens powder in your smoothie or morning routine.
- A morning snack to keep your energy and sugar level up.
- Protein and fat at lunch again, to maintain alertness. Lunch should be your largest meal because it is when your digestion peaks. Protein supplies the raw materials needed for a state of alertness and activity.
- An afternoon snack to support your afternoon energy level.
- Some protein and carbs at night—carbohydrates facilitate relaxation.
- Dinner should be your smallest meal, as it is when your digestion is slowing down.
- More carbohydrates in the summer and less in winter.
- Local and in-season food as much as possible—especially vegetables, to get the invaluable benefits of the phytonutrients.

I hope that you will continue to eat a protein-rich breakfast smoothie (if this has worked for you). Make lunch your biggest meal of the day, fill it with colors. Eat a dinner that has some protein, greens, and a healthy grain. It is the quality of the nutrients that is important and not whether the food is low-fat or low-carb. Get good-quality carbs and fat into you. These nutrient-dense foods are good for your genes and will help you feel less Spent. It is my greatest wish that you will continue to move your diet closer and closer to nature, eating more wild fish, grass-fed meats, and organic Spent Superfoods. I want you to eat less and less gluten, high-mercury fish, factory-farmed meats, soy, GMO foods, junk food, and, of course, sugar. The cleaner your diet, the better you will feel and the easier it will be to maintain your rhythm. For an ongoing conversation and connection to a community dedicated to staying un-Spent, go to www.spentmd.com.

SHOULD I KEEP TAKING THE SPENT SUPPLEMENTS?

This depends upon you. In my opinion, you should absolutely continue to take a greens powdered drink and a good multivitamin with B complex in the morning. The more carbs you eat, the more B vitamins you need (take them both morning and night if necessary). You should continue taking fish oil. It is also an invaluable resource for your body. So, yes, keep taking it in the morning.

As for the adaptogens, you can continue taking them for up to three months, and then I would suggest taking one month off. Remember: they are tonics, so they are most helpful to your body's system in the morning.

If your digestive tract is functioning better, you don't necessarily need to take probiotics all the time. My general recommendation is to have patients take them for a six- to eight-week course and then stop. Reintroduce them again in a month or two, allowing the body to build up its own natural flora. Then use them as a backup. Of course, if you have taken a course of antibiotics, it is always good to take probiotics afterward to rebuild the good bacteria in the gastrointestinal tract after it has been wiped out by antibiotics.

If the nighttime formula has been working for you, you can continue to take it. It should include calming amino acids that form inhibitory neurotransmitters (e.g., 5-HTP, GABA, and L-theanine). Taking calcium and magnesium at night can also help relaxation.

And if the CoQ10, carnitine, or alpha-lipoic acid has been making a difference in your energy levels, you can continue to take them. I personally take all these nutrients to stay healthy and prevent Spent. If you have other medical problems, you may also need more targeted supplementation. Go to my supplement section at www.spentmd.com.

Should I Continue to Do Restorative Exercise or Return to My Former Workout Schedule?

As I have tried to emphasize, restorative exercise trains the body to relax and recover. In our culture, the way most of us exercise is often stressful for the body and can promote that Spent feeling. This said, everyone's body is different and needs different forms of exercise to feel good. The kind of interval training you've been doing—in which you alternate between fast and slow periods—is my recommendation for how to continue after restorative exercise. But, if you feel strong and ready for a long run, do it, knowing that if you continually push your body too much and don't let it recover, you will get Spent. Likewise, if you now go back to being a couch potato, you can also end up Spent. So my general prescription for exercise and physical fitness is this:

Find a way to raise your heart rate four to five times a week, giving yourself at least one day to rest. Walk fast, jog, swim, or bike for at least 30 minutes, preferably with restorative or interval-type training. What time of day you exercise may be an important factor in how your exercise makes you feel. For most people, afternoon or early evening works best and is a great transition, moving from the busy workday into a relaxing night. However, if the morning works best for you or is more practical, do exercise in the morning.

Take every opportunity to move. Take the stairs. Walk to work. Park farther from the market.

Keep your core strong. Continue to do a few core-strengthening exercises at least three or four times a week. And any exercise program should also include stretching and some strength training, especially as you get older.

Have postural awareness. Continue to notice if you are slumping over your keyboard or always favoring one leg. Do core-strengthening exercises and hip, neck, back, and shoulder releases to fight chair body at least once or twice a week. They take so little time and make a profound difference.

Periodically get a massage or keep doing the release exercises with the foam roller and tennis balls.

If it has been helpful to you, continue to incorporate the restorative yoga into your nightly routine. The more you do it, the more benefits you will receive. Restorative poses like Supta Baddha Konasana (page 147) offer great premenstrual and menstrual relief. If you have really enjoyed the yoga in this book, you may want to check out a local yoga or Pilates class or buy a video to continue learning and exploring. I think Rodney Yee's and Patricia Waldon's video series are both excellent. Go to www.spentmd .com for more exercises and restorative yoga.

BEYOND DIET, SUPPLEMENTS, AND EXERCISE, WHAT SHOULD I DO?

Continue finding ways to help yourself chill out. Take breathing breaks during work. Remember, your breath is one of the key rhythms in your body. As I have mentioned, if you are struggling to bring your attention to your breath, the One Global Breath goggles and the One Breath Meditation at www.spentmd.com are great aids. When you relax and breathe slowly, it will always help.

In addition to the restorative yoga, establish a regular meditation or moving meditation practice (yoga, tai chi, dance). These are wonderful when it comes to stress management. They also help us become present to where we are in time and space, helping us rein in our wandering minds.

Do things that make you feel happy, laugh, and ease up, such as going to a funny movie with a friend or listening to music. By the way, there are some great CDs out now that help reset your brain waves. I have my patients listen to them while they have acupuncture treatments, with excellent results. Go to www .spentmd.com for music recommendations.

Continue limiting your exposure to toxins. The more environmentally and human-friendly you make your life, the less burden your body—particularly your hormones—will have to shoulder. To find out how you can do more to decrease your toxic load, go to www.spentmd.com.

Continue to integrate and play with the sleep tips I've given you. Good sleep habits are essential to restoring and maintaining rhythm. This means continuing to:

- *Get up at about the same time every day, regardless of how much sleep you get on a particular night. It is one of the most effective ways to keep your body rhythms in tune.*
- *Take a nap in the early afternoon if you need to. A siesta is not some out-there idea—it mirrors the body's need to rest after its biggest meal.*
- *Turn off your electronics by 10 p.m.*
- *Make sure that your bedroom is dark and cool.*
- *Get more sleep in the winter. This reflects the seasons' natural cycles. In the winter, the nights are longer, so getting more sleep mirrors our genetic blueprint for cold weather and shorter days.*

Get at least 30 minutes of sunlight daily, obviously not at peak hours. There is no replacement for sunlight. Our body clock responds to a variety of cues in our environment, the strongest of which is light. A pulse of sufficiently bright light at the appropriate time can affect our body clock and rhythms. If you don't get enough light, light therapy is helpful.[2]

Spend as much time as possible surrounded by trees, in the mountains, and by the ocean. Your body will entrain to the natural rhythms. The more time you can spend in nature, the better your rhythms will be. I know it sounds New Agey, but it is true.

Expand your joy and be more playful. You can do all of the above and still feel Spent if you don't have joy in your life. Happiness is truly the fire for our heads and hearts. It lights us up. Pema Chodron, one of my favorite writers and spiritual teachers, writes, "Always maintain only a joyful mind might sound like an impossible aspiration. As one man said to me, 'Always is a very long time.' Yet as we train in unblocking our hearts, we'll find that every moment contains the free-flowing openness and warmth that characterize unlimited joy."

Find meaning or purpose in your life. Find a cause or something outside yourself and your everyday life where you think you can make a difference or want to get involved with. As Friedrich Nietzsche said, "He who has a why to live for, can bear with almost any how." Having a sense of a higher purpose is an amazing natural high and probably one of the most potent factors in preventing Spent.

GET ON YOUR WAVE

Finding and keeping your rhythm is a lot like surfing. It takes some effort to paddle, but then, when you catch the wave, you get an incredible surge of energy. Then, once you're on the wave, you have to ride it. This also takes effort, but it is more about sensitivity to the water rushing beneath you. You have to feel where the energy is. Moving with the force is what allows you to travel along the face. The more you understand the way the wave and water work, the less effort you need to exert. Likewise, when you get in sync with your rhythms, you are literally on the same wavelength as your body. Your brain feels easier, your body lighter and easier. You are in the flow. You feel your feet, your arms, your breath, and your heart. You are not Spent. You are completely, utterly, and totally *alive*.

Troubleshooting

In my experience, about 80 percent of my patients feel significantly better after the six-week program, while 20 percent need a little extra attention to jump-start their systems into rhythm. If you are not sleeping better or feeling considerably more energy, fewer aches, and less mental stress (yet have given yourself to the program completely), or if you have improved but think you can feel even better, this chapter is for you. This section of the book is devoted to giving those of you who need more help some in-depth tools and information to help you solve your case of Spent.

The Spent program was developed to improve function of the various organ systems and treat the underlying imbalances that are usually involved when people are Spent. But sometimes specific areas need more targeted therapy and a significant boost to get them back into rhythm. Though everyone is different and has specific needs, in my experience, the 20 percent of my patients who do need more support generally need to have a complete panel of blood tests done and then act accordingly. Here's the protocol to follow:

First, get a workup from your doctor to rule out sleep apnea, anemia, and other problems that may be causing you to feel Spent. In addition to the regular blood panel, ask your doctor to order the following tests (these are regular tests that could be extremely helpful if you are Spent but are not routinely done):

25 OH vitamin D level (25-hydroxy vitamin D)
DHEA-S

A complete thyroid panel, including all of the following:
    Thyroid-stimulating hormone (TSH)
    Free T4 (free thyroxine)
    Free T3 (free triiodothyronine)
    Reverse T3
    Antithyroglobulin antibodies (anti-TG)
    Antithyroid peroxidase antibodies (anti-TPO)

Please note that the traditional bloods drawn to rule out thyroid problems are inadequate; a complete thyroid panel needs to be done. More than likely, you will have to tell your doctor that you want these specific tests included.

I know that this does not sound nearly as fun as doing a restorative yoga pose for ten minutes before bed or as easy as turning down the heat in your bedroom, but if you are still reading this and don't feel great, having these tests done and following next few steps are probably worth your while—and, I hope, will be the solution to feeling Spent.

Once you have the test results back, here is what to do:

1. If your vitamin D level is below 50ng/ml, take at least 2,000 IUs of vitamin D3 daily. And know that this means you are not getting enough sun! So it's also a good idea to make a real effort to get outside and feel the sun on your face (not at peak hours). Recheck your vitamin D level in three to four months.

2. If your DHEA is below 100, you may want to try taking a DHEA supplement. But before starting DHEA, I recommend trying some licorice root *if your blood pressure is low.* Licorice root is almost the perfect antidote for tired adrenals (a common cause of Spent and low DHEA). So if your blood pressure is low and you haven't already incorporated this into your program, take licorice root extract (*Glycyrrhiza glabra*) (standardized to 25% [150 milligrams] glycyrrhizic acid) twice a day. If you don't feel better after four weeks, you can see if DHEA is more helpful. As I said

when we first talked about licorice, *do not take licorice root if you have normal or high blood pressure.*

DHEA is the most common steroid hormone in the body. It is produced mainly by the adrenal glands and, to a lesser extent, elsewhere in the body (including fat cells). DHEA is metabolized from pregnenolone, the body's "master hormone," which itself is metabolized from cholesterol. DHEA can be metabolized into other sex hormones, including testosterone and the estrogens, and up to 150 individual metabolites. Sufficient levels of DHEA are required to ensure that your body can produce the hormones it needs when necessary. When DHEA levels are low, your body will not have enough of the precursors to many of the hormones necessary for optimal function.

From a cellular perspective, DHEA stimulates the mitochondria (which, as you now know, are the energy powerhouse of the cell) and is necessary for the production of energy. It is also vital to burning fat, and that is why along with fatigue, elderly individuals often gain weight and often store the fat gained in the abdominal region. DHEA levels drop dramatically as people age. Young adults have almost unlimited energy (and high DHEA levels); elderly people have relatively little. And although there are many factors in why you are Spent, a lack of DHEA may be the missing key. There are also pronounced differences in the average DHEA levels of men and women, with women on average having lower DHEA levels.

If you are going to take DHEA, I suggest you do it under the care of your doctor. Ideally, DHEA replacement therapy should begin with blood testing to establish a base range. Generally the suggested starting dosage of DHEA is 25 to 50 milligrams for men and 5 to 10 milligrams for women, taken in the morning before breakfast. Optimally you want your DHEA level to be 250 to 500 µg/dL for males and 150 to 350 µg/dL for females.

Important: After four to six weeks, another test is recommended to measure serum DHEA. All individuals react differently to DHEA replacement therapy, so it's a good idea to closely monitor your blood levels and side effects.

Special Cautions:

- *Because DHEA may be converted into estrogen, women with breast, uterine, or ovarian cancer are advised not to begin DHEA therapy, which may increase the severity of their cancer. Healthy women taking DHEA should also monitor their blood levels of estrogen and free testosterone to make sure that DHEA is not affecting these other sex hormones detrimentally.*

- *Men should not begin DHEA therapy before having their prostate-specific antigen (PSA) levels tested and undergoing a digital rectal exam, to measure the size and consistency of the prostate. Men with prostate cancer or severe benign prostate disease are advised to avoid DHEA because it can be converted into testosterone, which may promote cell proliferation or cause an increase in dihydrotestosterone (DHT). To make sure DHEA is tolerated, men should consider having their DHEA blood levels tested initially after three months and then every six or twelve months, along with their levels of free testosterone, estrogen, and DHT.*

- *Do not take DHEA if you could be pregnant, are breast-feeding, or could have prostate, breast, uterine, or ovarian cancer. DHEA can cause androgenic effects in women, such as acne, deepening of the voice, facial hair growth, and hair loss.*

3. Even if your blood tests are normal and you still have the following symptoms:

Fatigue
Sluggishness
Aches and pains
A low sex drive
Dry, scaly skin that is not improving
Coarse, brittle, dry hair that may be falling out
Depression that is not improving
Constipation that is not improving
Weight gain or difficulty losing weight in spite of being on
    the Spent program

Fluid retention or puffiness that is not improving
Muscle aches and weakness that are not improving
Intolerance to the cold that is not improving
Decreased sweating

you may have low thyroid function and the diet and nutrients in the Spent program may not have been enough to optimize it, and you may need to be more aggressive about dealing with your low thyroid function. Please understand that thyroid function tests have inherent limitations, so this means you need to use them as only one part of your assessment. It is vital to know that even a comprehensive panel of blood tests may not always show thyroid dysfunction. This is why thyroid dysfunction often goes undetected because, as you see, a lot of these symptoms are vague and pretty common.

There are three ways to assess thyroid function:

Symptoms
Underarm temperature
Blood test results that indicate that the thyroid is off

While you are waiting for your thyroid blood test results, measure your basal temperature. It is normally recommended that you take your temperature in the armpit first thing in the morning—without much movement—for 10 minutes. Record it for 5 to 7 days in a row. Menopausal women and men can take their temperature any day. Women of child-bearing age need to take it beginning on day two or three of their menstrual cycle due to hormonal fluctuations. If the temperature is below 97.0, that could be an indication of hypothyroidism. If you have normal blood tests yet have the classic symptoms of thyroid dysfunction and a temperature below 97.0, you more than likely have an imbalance.

This is because the blood tests measure how much thyroid hormone is in the blood and not how much is getting to the tissues. Thyroid dysfunction can occur when there is peripheral cellular resistance to thyroid hormone or when there is a problem with the conversion of T4 (inactive hormone) to T3 (active hormone). People with cellular resistance may have perfectly normal circulating thyroid hormone levels but still have signs and symptoms of hypothyroidism. Work with your doctor to interpret your thyroid tests properly. You cannot be passive. When it is not absolutely black-and-white clear that a patient has a thyroid problem, most doctors need to be pushed to look at the gray. So be an advocate for yourself.

The traditional way to diagnose hypothyroidism is when your thyroid-stimulating hormone (TSH) is elevated beyond the normal reference range. For most labs, this is about 5.0. TSH is secreted by the pituitary gland when it senses there is not enough thyroid hormone in the bloodstream. It is part of the body's feedback system to maintain stable amounts of the thyroid hormones thyroxine (T4) and triiodothyronine (T3) in the blood. If your TSH is over 5.0, you will be diagnosed with hypothyroidism, but unfortunately this is not sensitive enough. Most practitioners who work with thyroid dysfunction feel that the upper limit of normal for TSH should be 2.0 and not 5.0. So if your TSH is above 2.0, there is a good chance you have thyroid dysfunction.

In addition to the TSH, you should ask your doctor to measure your free T4 and free T3 levels. Free T3 and free T4 levels are the only accurate measures of the actual active thyroid hormone levels in the blood. If these are low, even if your TSH is below 2.0, you should also consider being more aggressive about treating your thyroid dysfunction if you still feel Spent. Fairly often, the TSH is normal, free T4 is normal, and free T3 is low. This means that there is a problem with the conversion of T4 to T3.

Work with your doctor to treat your thyroid dysfunction properly. Again, partner with him or her to solve and treat your case.

Once a diagnosis of hypothyroidism has been made, and it has been decided that you need thyroid replacement therapy, you will once again need to work with your doctor to choose the right one for you. Most people will need to combine the inactive T4 hormone levothyroxine (found in Synthroid, Levothroid, and

Levoxyl) and the active hormone T3 (found in Cytomel). It is essential that the correct type of replacement therapy in the right dose be given. Most conventional doctors routinely prescribe Synthroid for hypothyroidism. This may be fine for some patients, but for many it does not work. This is because levothyroxine or T4 (Synthroid is synthetic T4) is not the active thyroid hormone; T3 is. And if your body is not converting T4 to T3, you will not be getting the active hormone. In fact, for some people, giving them Synthroid may actually even make them feel worse, because although most T3 is made from converting T4 to T3 in the liver, the thyroid gland does produce some T3, and its production decreases in the presence of increased thyroxine.

Also, when you are Spent, you have usually been under a lot of stress and have not been getting the right amount of necessary nutrients to optimize your thyroid function. This often leads to problems converting T4 to the active hormone T3, so just giving T4, as when giving Synthroid, is usually not appropriate for Spent patients.

So I suggest you ask your physician to start you on one of the three natural thyroid replacements, which are Armour, Westhroid, and Naturethroid. They are all made from frozen porcine glands and there are minor differences between the three, but they all have both T4 and T3 together. In a 1999 study published in *The New England Journal of Medicine,* patients with hypothyroidism showed greater improvements in mood and brain function if they received Armour thyroid rather than Synthroid (thyroxine).[1] It is important to remember that T3 has a short half-life. That means a once-a-day dosage is not enough. You will need to take it twice a day, preferably on an empty stomach because protein, calcium, and iron are known to interfere with the absorption of the hormone.

If you do start thyroid hormone replacement, it is essential to start at the lowest dosage. If, after taking that dose for two weeks, you are not better, double the dosage for two weeks and then reassess. This slow increase in the dose will ensure the most adequate dosage with no side effects or hyperthyroid reaction from overdosage.

4. If you are still having digestive problems or you have the following symptoms:

Bloating
Gas
Indigestion
Reflux
Abnormal bowel movements
Abdominal pain or discomfort

you may need more targeted treatment for the gastrointestinal tract, taking all of these additional supplements for the best results:

An herbal "antibiotic"
A glutamine-based formula to restore the lining of the gut
More probiotics
Digestive enzymes with meals
A fiber formula

Go to www.spentmd.com or see my last book, *Total Renewal,* for more information. The two most common causes of continued digestive dysfunction are (1) not enough good bacteria, which may lead to an overgrowth of bad bacteria, yeast, or parasites or to bad bacteria moving into areas where they shouldn't be, for instance the small intestine, and (2) a breaking down of the thin lining of the gastrointestinal wall, leading to a leaky gut and Spent. The herbal "antibiotic" formula removes the bad bacteria, the probiotic formula repopulates the good flora in your gut, the glutamine-based formula helps the body heal a leaky or poor gut lining, and the digestive enzymes help to break down and digest food.

If you would like to be clear about exactly what your body might need, functional testing (see below) is indicated. The best noninvasive diagnostic test for digestive problems is a comprehensive stool analysis, which can help target specific treatments. Both

Metametrix (www.metametrix.com) and Genova Diagnostics (www.gdx.net) do these tests, which check for parasites, yeast, and abnormal bacteria (and see if you have enough good bacteria), as well as exploring risk factors for more serious gastrointestinal problems such as colorectal cancer.

5. Doing a more intensive cleanse may kick-start your system. Go to www.spentmd.com for more information on how to do this.

6. If you are not better, all of the traditional and above-discussed tests are normal, and you have tried all of the above suggestions (and probably more), it may be necessary to have some functional testing done as well.

Functional tests are not standard medical tests. Functional testing goes to the next level of investigating the biochemical and metabolic imbalances and dysfunctions likely to cause a specific disease process or suboptimal functioning. But like standard tests, they still measure the imbalances using your blood, urine, stool, and saliva.

As we talked about early on, standard medical testing—as in traditional Western medicine addresses acute or advanced organic diseases. So, although you may have had the symptoms of Spent for months or even years and still feel sick, the chances are that the results of your standard tests are normal because they are screening for a particular ailment or pathology.

The difference between functional tests and standard tests is that functional tests assess organ "function" as opposed to organ "pathology." Functional testing identifies the many physiological precursors that lead to chronic conditions, including Spent, whereas standard medical testing will find abnormalities only if there is pathology or imbalance in the tissues or organs already. It does not pick up dysfunction, which will predate a pathology. Because everyone has a unique biochemistry based on many factors, such as genetics, lifestyle, diet, environmental exposure to chemicals, and psychological and physical stresses, an imbalance that may not be a big deal to many people's bodies might be tremendous for yours. And rather than looking for a particular disease, functional testing looks at what is throwing your body off—or where the dysfunction is.

I discussed the comprehensive stool analysis above as a way of investigating digestive dysfunctions, but if you are Spent, functional testing can also help identify:

Cellular energy dysfunction
Nutritional deficiencies
Adrenal exhaustion/dysfunction
Hormone imbalances
Heavy-metal toxicity
Sleep disorders
Liver detoxification dysfunctions
Food intolerances and allergies

All of the above could be factors in why you are Spent. Functional testing requires that you work closely with a health care professional trained in functional medicine to resolve the problems identified. Unless your doctor practices functional medicine, he or she will be unfamiliar with these tests and may consider them to be hocus pocus. If you have a good relationship with your doctor, ask him or her to indulge you and order the tests. Explain that these tests can be enormously helpful and can detect problems long before more traditional tests find anything wrong. Say that these tests are complements to the usual testing that traditional physicians use. Blame me, and suggest that your doctor consult the functional medicine Web site (www.functionalmedicine .org). If you don't love your doctor and trust him or her, perhaps it is time for you to find another physician whom you feel you can trust and who will really be a partner in your healing. If you have come this far and gone to every length you can think of to heal, you really do need help and someone to champion your cause. You can find a list of trained functional medicine practitioners at www.functionalmedicine.org.

If your doctor does not know of any labs that do functional tests, there is a list of them in the Resources section (page 305). Many labs around the country have developed a number of amazing assessment tools that allow practitioners to determine a patient's functional status. Many of these tests are reimbursed by insurance companies, but I suggest you ask your physician and/or staff about reimbursement before you proceed with testing. Some tests may need to be paid for out of pocket, and some are not allowed in certain states, particularly New York.

Of all the functional tests, the one that is simplest and that I find most helpful as a basic "starter" test is the urine Organix Profile test by Metametrix. All it needs is a first morning urine sample, which is easy to do. It is a good all-around screening test for Spent, as it is basically a cellular energy profile, testing your mitochondrial function, but it also provides important information in the areas of:

Vitamin and mineral insufficiencies
Insufficiency of amino acids such as carnitine and NAC
Oxidative damage and antioxidant sufficiency
Detoxification sufficiency
B-complex deficiency
Mitochondrial energy production (via citric acid cycle
    components)
Lipoic acid and CoQ10 sufficiency
Specific dysbiosis markers for bacterial and yeast overgrowth

The Organix Profile provides insight into the body's cellular metabolic processes and the efficiency of metabolic function. Identifying metabolic blocks that can be treated nutritionally allows individual tailoring of interventions that maximize patients' responses and lead to improved outcomes. Organic acids are metabolic intermediates produced in pathways of central energy production, detoxification, neurotransmitter breakdown, or intestinal microbial activity. Accumulation of certain organic acids in the urine often signals a metabolic inhibition or block. This may be due to a nutrient deficiency, an inherited enzyme deficit, toxic buildup, or drug effect. The profile evaluates organic acids that play a key role in the generation of cellular energy. It can uncover the important metabolic imbalances associated with Spent. For more information, go to www.metametrix.com/content/ DirectoryOfServices/0291OrganixBasic-Urine. This process of working to refine your thyroid, adrenals, digestion, and detoxification systems and anything else that is throwing your balance off takes time—often months. It can be hard, annoying, stressful, upsetting, thrilling, relieving, and healing all at the same time. I'd encourage you to stay with it.

You Will Heal

My patient Sue had been through the health wringer—several bouts of cancer, having her thyroid removed, chronic bronchitis. For a while, it seemed as if it was never going to stop.

For years, Sue had gotten used to feeling less than great. And, as she tells it, "The stuff that didn't feel right was subtle. For example, every time I saw the eye doctor, I told him it just felt like my vision was wrong, and he would explain that I was getting older. And it seemed like I was just getting more and more tired. And bigger."

But then last summer, her husband, as she says, "took his life into his hands" and told her that she was . . . fat. Sue says that initially she was too tired even to care. But then even she noticed that her clothes were getting a bit snug. Having seen me before, Sue put herself on the Spent restorative diet plan, giving up sugar, caffeine, gluten, and processed foods. She exercised—walking and doing yoga—but dragged herself through it. She lost some weight, but compared to a normal person's response to this diet and exercise regime, it was nothing.

She also noticed that her skin was dry, her usually strong nails were peeling, and her hair was brittle. She drank aloe vera and poured on more and more creams to soften her skin. Meanwhile, she was freezing even in the intense heat of a New York City summer. Her husband said her preferred temperature at home was more suitable for orchid growing than human living.

She described her head and body as feeling as if everything was a little gray. It was a fight to get started in the morning and a fight to want to do anything. She had forgotten what it was like to move with energy. Everything she did was the result of will and discipline. Her speech was a little garbled, and words came out wrong. There was no point in pressing the gas pedal because there was no gas.

It is hard also because when you feel like Sue, you start to do what you can to get moving. Sue was up to nine double espressos (and chocolate!) a day to write her second book. And she kept looking to food to be a stimulant because—she needed a stimulant. It is a vicious cycle—the less energy she had, the less she could take care of herself.

Sue asked her general practitioner to check her thyroid because she had had her thyroid removed years before and knew that some of the symptoms she was having could mean she was hypothyroid. The doctor ran the regular screens and told Sue she was normal. But Sue felt anything but normal.

If she had a big meeting with clients on a Tuesday, she would try to get to whatever city she needed to be in by Monday afternoon so she could stay in bed and rest until the meeting. This way she would have an hour and a half of juice in the battery.

After several of these business trips, she came back to my office and had me do a thorough check of her thyroid. I discovered that although she was on Synthroid, she was not converting the Synthroid (T4) to the active thyroid hormone T3. All I did was add Cytomel (T3) to her regimen. Within a few hours of taking the medicine, Sue's vision was better. Within a day, she claims, she was literally "dancing" around New York.

In an e-mail to me, Sue described exactly what we have been talking about throughout the book, "Most doctors are great about fixing what is wrong. They don't seem to care so much about what it takes to feel truly well, or value the pursuit of that as a goal. Sometimes they make it seem selfish and spoiled to want that, although I now know that I really can't be there for other people, or do any of the things I am meant to do, unless I am well. This tiny thyroid malfunction absolutely limited my life and the new medication means literally that I have a new life. I have no idea what I will do once I have energy in the afternoon and evening as well."

My point is that healing takes time and energy (when we sometimes have none), but it does happen, and I know that if you stick with it, it will happen for you.

PART IV

Eating to Relieve Spent

A Personal Note from Janice

With so many wonderful cookbooks available, you may be wondering why we have chosen to include a recipe section in a health book. But while there are endless amazing and delicious recipes available—in cookbooks and on the Web—many of them call for dairy or gluten or soy, which you are taking a break from while on the Spent restorative eating program. And, although Frank and I do occasionally have cheese and pasta, we cook and eat primarily in line with the Spent restorative eating program—and have for years. So we thought it might be helpful to offer you a look at some of the foods and methods we use, more as an example of how to cook on the restorative eating plan than a recipe-driven diet to follow.

Our way of cooking and eating is a philosophy motivated by our desire to eat in a way that really feeds our bodies and makes us feel good, including not spending hours in the kitchen, which can be as exhausting as anything else.

Every week we go to the market and stock up on loads of Spent Superfoods: fresh herbs, a wide assortment of fresh vegetables and fruits (including frozen fruits for smoothies), some low-mercury fish, organic free-range eggs, grass-fed beef, and organic free-range chicken. When we get home, we spend some time together chopping and organizing all of the vegetables so that our refrigerator becomes a giant salad and fruit bar that we can use all week. Our fridge is stocked with glass containers full of baby spinach and salad greens, sliced carrots, peppers, cauliflower and broccoli cut into florets, butternut squash already cut into small cubes, diced celery, sliced mushrooms, and shredded cabbage. Every morning, we have our choice of fruits and berries for our smoothie. And every night we have the option of making a soup from the diced butternut squash, a stir-fry with chicken and Asian greens, or, if we're feeling like comfort foods, grilled steak, sautéed spinach, and roasted parsnips, which taste like sweet French fries. And if we have any leftovers, which we often do, we incorporate them into another meal, such as a big, colorful salad—so that we more often than not "make it once and use it twice." If you are wondering exactly how much time cooking like this takes, please know that when I mean I don't want to spend time in the kitchen, I mean not much more than 30 minutes. This is why all of the recipes I've included take approximately 30 minutes (except for the roasted vegetables such as the parsnips, which take 45 minutes and need little attention).

This is why the first section, "Foods for Renewal," is not recipes, it is an even more thorough list of vegetables and ingredients than the one in the "Prepare" section of the book. *You do not have to buy all of these foods at once.* This is simply the complete list of Spent Superfoods and sanctioned foods that Frank believes are best for healing Spent. This said, you want to have enough fruits, vegetables, and protein sources on hand that you can come home and whip up a stir-fry or a salad and not have the extra burden of going to the market and chopping more than once or twice (if you like really fresh vegetables) a week. As Frank said in the Prepare Section, having food that is ready to go from fridge to pot is the key to cooking when you are Spent. Once you get the hang of stocking your fridge and approaching cooking in this way, you will find that it is timesaving and liberating and might even unleash your inner Julia Child. For your convenience, I've also put this list online at www.spentmd.com for you to download and take with you to the market. Of course, all of this is to encourage you to think "out of the box and canned" and into the fresh and whole in an easy, delicious, and nutritious way. After what will seem like an encyclopedia of fruits, vegetables, and foods, you will arrive at the Recipes for Renewal section. We have divided the recipes up into three basic sections:

- *Breakfast foods*
- *Lunch and dinner foods, because these days these foods are so interchangeable*
- *Sweets and snacks*

With a few exceptions, most of the recipes are gluten-free, sugar-free, and dairy-free, and use low-mercury fish.

As Frank said in Daily Beat 2, breakfast is the most important meal for people who are Spent. While there are endless options for a phytonutrient-rich breakfast with healthy fats and oils that support your natural physiological rhythms and needs, this is our selection of what we believe are the best Spent-healing ways to nourish yourself in the morning. As you know, Frank loves smoothies, and so do I. So we've included recipes for banana smoothies, berry smoothies, avocado smoothies, and no-blender-necessary smoothies. But recognizing that not everyone embraces the blender the way we do, we've also included a few breakfast options for those who are not smoothie fans or want something warm for breakfast.

Our lunch and dinners are completely devoted to the three main eating concepts that Frank talks about in the six-week program: add as much phytonutrient-rich color to your diet as you can, eat according to the physiological rhythm and needs of your body—bigger lunch, more modest dinner—and eat what is local and in season. So we've included meals that use massive amounts of color—red, yellow, orange, green, purple, white; understand that you want a simple dinner—for example, a salad with nuts and a bit of goat cheese with some soup; and consider that your body needs warmer, heartier foods in the winter and more carbohydrates in the summer. This way, no matter what season it is, you will find foods here to make and eat.

Finally, because we know everyone needs a treat now and then, we've included some sugar-free, dairy-free, gluten-free sweets that are so good that you will not miss your cookie jar. I've also included a few snack suggestions to further support your rhythm eating—what Frank calls a "snack attack"—the two smaller meals that you should be eating so that your blood sugar doesn't drop between meals.

My sincere hope is that all of this will make your restorative eating program easy, nutritious, and inspiring. At our house, eating is a celebration of family, friends, and the season and of caring for our bodies. As George Bernard Shaw says, "There is no love sincerer than the love of food."

So let's get to the food!

Foods for Renewal

First comes the list of Spent Superfoods and other great foods to eat to help you heal from Spent. Please note that we have not included only vegetables and fruits that correspond with our recipes. This is a comprehensive guideline for healthier eating. For a downloadable list of all four food groups, go to www.spentmd.com.

EAT AS MUCH AS YOU LIKE

Spent Superfoods are highlighted in *italics*.

Vegetables
Asparagus	Mushrooms
Avocado (actually a fruit)	*Mustard greens*
Bok choy	*Olives*
Broccoli	Onions
Broccoli rabe	*Sea Vegetables*
Brussels sprouts	*Spinach*
Cabbage (green and red)	Sprouts
Carrots	*Swiss chard*
Cauliflower	*Tomatoes (actually a fruit)*
Celery	*Watercress*
Chinese cabbage	Alfalfa sprouts
Collard greens	Artichokes
Dandelion greens	Arugula
Kale	Beets

Beet greens
Butternut squash
Chicory
Chives
Cucumbers
Eggplant
Endive
Escarole
Fennel
Horseradish
Jerusalem artichoke
Jicama
Kohlrabi
Leeks
Lettuce: romaine, red leaf, green
    leaf

Okra
Parsnips
Peppers (hot): cayenne, chile,
    jalapeño
Peppers (sweet): red, green,
    yellow
Pumpkin
Radishes
Rutabagas
Squash (winter and summer)
Sweet potato
Turnips
Yams
Zucchini

Fruits

Apples
Apricots
Blackberries
Blueberries
Cantaloupes
Cherries
Coconut
Cranberries
Figs (fresh)
Goji berries
Grapefruit
Grapes
Guava (fresh)
Honeydew melon
Kiwi fruit

Lemons
Limes
Mangoes
Nectarines
Papayas
Peaches
Pears
Persimmons
Pineapples
Pomegranates
Raspberries
Star fruits
Strawberries
Watermelon

Nuts and Seeds

Nuts should be raw and unsalted. As mentioned in the "Prepare" section, if you like roasted nuts, you can slow-roast them in your toaster oven at 160 to 175° F. for 15 to 20 minutes.

Almonds	Hazelnuts
Brazil nuts	Macadamia nuts
Ground flaxseeds	Pine nuts
Pecans	Pistachio nuts
Walnuts	Pumpkin seeds
Almond butter	Sesame seeds
Cashews	Sunflower seeds
Chestnuts	Tahini (sesame paste)

Beans and Legumes

Beans (all types)	Lentils
Chickpeas (garbanzo beans)	Peas: green and snow
Edamame (green soybeans)	
Fermented soy (natto, tempeh, and miso)	

Fish

Anchovies	*Canned sardines in olive oil*
Black cod (sablefish)	*Wild salmon (fresh and canned)*

Poultry and Meat

Beef (grass-fed)	Turkey (free-range and organic)
Chicken (free-range and organic)	Wild game (buffalo, venison, elk, ostrich)
Lamb (grass-fed)	
Pork (grass-fed)	

Eggs and Dairy Substitutes

Organic eggs (Note: It is best to cook the yolk whole—poached or boiled)	Almond milk (unsweetened)
	Other nut milks (unsweetened)
Whey protein powder (vanilla or plain)	

Herbs, Spices, and Condiments (fresh, ground, or dried)

Cilantro (coriander)	Curry powder
Cinnamon	Dill
Garlic	Garam masala
Ginger	Mint
Oregano	Mustard
Turmeric	Paprika
Arrowroot (thickener)	Parsley
Basil	Pepper: black and cayenne
Cardamom	Rosemary
Chili peppers (red)	Sage
Cloves	Sea salt (coarse and fine)
Cumin	Thyme

Vinegar

Apple cider vinegar	Rice wine vinegar
Balsamic vinegar	White wine vinegar
Red wine vinegar	

Specialty Foods

Barley grass	*Wheat grass*
Chlorella	*Wild blue-green algae*
Spirulina	

EAT IN MODERATION

Spent-sanctioned foods; eat a maximum of one to two servings a day.

Fruits and Vegetables

Bananas	Raisins
Oranges	Potatoes
Prunes	

Grains

Amaranth (fairly high in protein)	Brown rice pasta
Brown rice	Buckwheat

Ezekiel bread
Millet
Oats: steel-cut or pure oats
    (even though oats are a
    gluten grain)

Quinoa (fairly high in protein)

Poultry and Meat

Always try to buy grass-fed, antibiotic-free, organic meat if possible. If it is not, use skinless lean cuts of factory-farmed chicken, turkey, beef, veal, or pork, all trimmed of any visible fat, for example, lean beef and pork or chicken and turkey breasts. I do not recommend eating the following fish or factory-farmed meats more than twice a week.

Fish and Shellfish

Bass (striped)
Blue crab (mid-Atlantic)
Catfish
Char
Clams
Croaker
Flounder
Haddock
King salmon (smoked)
Light tuna (canned)

Mussels
Oysters
Rainbow trout
Scallops
Shrimp (domestic)
Sole (Pacific)
Squid (calamari)
Sturgeon
Tilapia

Dairy Products, Dairy Substitutes, and Eggs

Although some of the following are made from cow's milk, yogurt and the cheeses are easier to digest.

Butter (organic)
Cheese: goat's milk and sheep's
    milk
Cottage cheese
Farmer's cheese
Feta cheese
Kefir

Milk (organic and raw)
Rice milk (unsweetened)
Ricotta cheese
Yogurt: goat's milk and sheep's
    milk
Yogurt (plain organic unsweet-
    ened)

Specialty Foods

Cacao nibs	Chocolate (dark)

Sweeteners

Agave syrup	Real maple syrup (small
Blackstrap molasses (small	amounts)
amounts)	Stevia
Raw unprocessed honey (small	Xylitol
amounts)	

AVOID FOR THE SIX WEEKS YOU ARE ON THE PROGRAM AND EAT ONLY SPARINGLY THEREAFTER

Eat a maximum of one serving a week after the program.

Poultry and Meat

Factory-farmed chicken, turkey,	Sausages
beef, veal, pork	

Fish and Shellfish

Albacore tuna (canned)	Oysters (Gulf Coast)
Bluefish	Pike
Cod	Pollack
Crab	Sea bass
Grouper (wild)	Shark
Halibut	Swordfish
Herring	Tilefish
King mackerel	Tuna steaks
Largemouth bass	Walleye
Lobster (Maine)	White croaker
Mahimahi	Whitefish
Marlin	

Beans and Legumes

Peanut butter

Peanuts (are legumes, not nuts)

Unfermented soy products, including all processed soy foods

Grains

Includes most breads, bagels, pastas, and most commercial breakfast cereals.

Barley

Bran

Corn

Couscous

Durum wheat

Farina

Farro

Kamut

Oats (unless pure oats)

Rye

Semolina

Spelt

Wheat (including whole wheat products)

Wheat germ

Dairy Products and Dairy Substitutes

Milk (including organic milk)

Milk products apart from those listed under "Eat in Moderation."

Other

Alcohol

Coffee

AVOID AS MUCH AS POSSIBLE

Sweeteners: high-fructose corn syrup, brown sugar, cane sugar, beet sugar, fructose, sucrose, glucose, maltose, dextrose, succinat, molasses, date sugar, grape sugar, corn syrup, corn sugar, fruit juice concentrate, sorbitol, barley malt, caramel, carob syrup

Artificial sweeteners: Aspartame (NutraSweet, Equal), saccharin (Sweet'N Low), sucralose (Splenda)

Artificial colorings: FD&C Red no. 3, Yellow nos. 5 and 6, Blue nos. 1 and 2

Artificial flavor enhancers: monosodium glutamate (MSG), yeast extract, hydrolyzed vegetable protein, autolyzed vegetable protein, textured protein, calcium caseinate, potassium bromate

Preservatives: sulfites, nitrites, nitrates, BHA, BHT, TBHQ

Hydrogenated or partially hydrogenated fats and oils

Processed foods, including frankfurters, hot dogs, lunch meats

Packaged foods

Sodas and diet sodas

Fruit juice (unless it is freshly squeezed)

Canned foods (exceptions are wild salmon, sardines in olive oil, organic beans, olives, and organic tomatoes)

Baked goods: cakes, cupcakes, pies, doughnuts, pastries, most desserts

Crackers, pretzels, and chips (all kinds)

Candy bars

Margarine

French fries and fried food in general

Most pasta and other commercial sauces (full of sugar or high-fructose corn syrup)

Many commercial salad dressings (frequently full of sugar and MSG)

Recipes for Renewal

Breakfast

For nonsmoothie mornings . . .

HOT CEREAL

Although I am not a huge fan, the permissible options while on the restorative eating program are slow-cooking oats, quinoa, and amaranth.

Cook the grains according to the instructions on the package, adding a little alcohol-free vanilla extract to the cooking water. When cooked, add ¼ cup chopped walnuts, a dash of cinnamon, and a little agave syrup to sweeten. 1 tablespoon ground flaxseed is also a nutritional extra. Serve with almond milk if desired.

RAW MUESLI   *serves 4*

8 ounces uncooked rolled oats
1 cup nut milk (almond or brazil nut)
1 tablespoon unsweetened shredded coconut
2 tablespoons chopped walnuts or almonds
2 tablespoons ground flaxseeds
2 tablespoons sesame seeds
2 tablespoons pumpkin seeds

8 ounces fresh berries
1 apple, peeled and grated

In a large bowl, mix together the oats, nut milk, shredded coconut, nuts, and seeds. Cover and place in the fridge overnight. In the morning, add berries and grated apple.

BREAKFAST PANINI

Layer 1 slice of sprouted Ezekiel bread with a couple of leaves of arugula. Add slices of avocado and tomato and drizzle with a little extra-virgin olive oil. Top with another slice of Ezekiel bread and toast in a panini press. When you are allowed dairy, try adding buffalo mozzarella cheese. (This can be an open sandwich too—it does not have to be toasted.)

SARDINES ON TOAST

Toast a slice of sprouted Ezekiel bread. Top with fresh arugula leaves, sardines (in olive oil, drained), and tomato slices. Sprinkle with sea salt and freshly ground pepper.

EGGS

2 boiled or poached organic eggs

Smoothies

My most favorite breakfast food. As Frank has said, smoothies are easy to prepare and a nutrient-dense meal. You will need a blender, preferably one that can crush ice.

GREENA-COLADA AVOCADO SMOOTHIE

1 cup frozen pineapple chunks
1 cup coconut water
$\frac{1}{4}$ avocado
1 serving or 3–4 tablespoons vanilla or plain whey protein powder
1 serving or 2 teaspoons greens powder
$\frac{1}{2}$–1 tablespoon coconut oil
4 ice cubes

Blend in a blender until smooth and creamy. If you cannot find coconut water, use $\frac{1}{2}$ cup nut milk, such as unsweetened almond milk, and $\frac{1}{2}$ cup filtered water.

GREENO MOJITO AVOCADO SMOOTHIE

$\frac{1}{4}$ avocado
1 serving or 3–4 tablespoons vanilla or plain whey protein powder
1 serving or 2 teaspoons greens powder
1 teaspoon vanilla extract
$\frac{1}{4}$ cup fresh mint leaves
Juice of one lime
1 tablespoon agave syrup
$\frac{3}{4}$ cup filtered water
3–4 ice cubes

Blend in a blender until smooth and creamy.

BLUEBERRY AVOCADO SMOOTHIE

1 cup frozen organic blueberries
$\frac{1}{4}$ avocado
1 cup coconut water
Juice of half a lime
1 tablespoon agave syrup
1 serving or 3–4 tablespoons vanilla or plain whey protein powder

1 serving or 2 teaspoons greens powder
4 ice cubes

Blend in a blender until smooth and creamy.

CHERRY PEACH AVOCADO SMOOTHIE

$\frac{1}{4}$ avocado
1 serving or 3–4 tablespoons vanilla or plain whey protein powder
1 serving or 2 teaspoons greens powder
1 cup filtered water
$\frac{1}{2}$ cup frozen organic cherries
$\frac{1}{2}$ cup frozen organic peaches
1 tablespoon agave syrup
Juice of $\frac{1}{2}$ lime
3–4 ice cubes

Blend in a blender until smooth and creamy.

The next selection of smoothies in this section can be made with either 2 tablespoons of raw nut butter (almond or sesame) plus 1 cup of water *or* ½ cup almond milk and ½ cup water and no raw nut butter. Blend until smooth.

If the smoothie is too thick, add more water. If you need to sweeten it, add 1–2 tablespoons of agave syrup.

PINEAPPLE PEACH BANANA SMOOTHIE

1 small frozen banana, cut into chunks
$\frac{1}{2}$ cup frozen pineapple pieces
$\frac{1}{2}$ cup frozen peach slices
$\frac{1}{2}$–1 teaspoon vanilla extract
1 serving or 3–4 tablespoons vanilla or plain whey protein powder
1 serving or 2 teaspoons greens powder
2 tablespoons raw unsalted almond butter

(continued on next page)

    1 tablespoon flaxseed oil
    1 cup filtered water
    4 ice cubes

Blend in a blender until smooth and creamy.

BANANA BERRY SMOOTHIE

    1 frozen small banana in chunks
    1 cup mixed frozen berries
    1 serving or 3–4 tablespoons vanilla or plain whey protein powder
    1 serving or 2 teaspoons greens powder
    ½ cup almond milk
    ½ cup filtered water
    4 ice cubes

Blend in a blender until smooth and creamy.

STRAWBERRY MANGO SENSATION

    ½ cup diced strawberries (fresh or frozen)
    ½ cup frozen mango chunks
    1 frozen small banana in chunks
    1 serving or 3–4 tablespoons vanilla or plain whey protein powder
    1 serving or 2 teaspoons greens powder
    ½ cup almond milk
    ½ cup filtered water
    4 ice cubes

Blend in a blender until smooth and creamy.

GINGER PEAR SMOOTHIE

    1 large ripe pear, peeled and diced (a Bartlett pear is best)
    1 frozen banana in chunks
    1 teaspoon vanilla extract

Pinch of ground ginger
Juice of $\frac{1}{2}$ lime
$\frac{1}{4}$ cup almond milk
$\frac{1}{2}$ cup filtered water
1 serving or 3–4 tablespoons vanilla or plain whey protein powder
1 serving or 2 teaspoons greens powder
3 ice cubes

Blend in a blender until smooth and creamy.

WORKDAY WONDER SMOOTHIE

The nonblender, fast and easy smoothie.

1 serving or 3–4 tablespoons vanilla or plain whey protein powder
1 serving or 2 teaspoons greens powder
1 serving or 2 teaspoons berry powder (optional)
$\frac{1}{2}$ cup almond milk
$\frac{1}{2}$ cup filtered water
Or 1 cup filtered water only

Place in shaker cup and shake until well blended.

Although not a thick smoothie, this one provides all the essential nutrients for a complete breakfast. It can also be made at work since the ingredients are in powder form, thereby eliminating the "I don't have time for breakfast" excuse.

Make Your Own Smoothie

I believe in the imagination. What I cannot see is infinitely
more important than what I can see.
—Duane Michaels

While I have offered you what seems like dozens of smoothie recipes, if you would like to experiment and come up with your own smoothie, here are the general guidelines for achieving the right balance of protein, smoothie texture, and taste. Here are the essentials.

Liquid: You will need about 1 cup liquid. You can use filtered water, coconut water (liquid drained from fresh baby coconuts; also available in small juice-box-size cartons), or nut milk. Nut milk such as almond milk can be store-bought; please choose unsweetened. I usually mix ½ cup nut milk and ½ cup water. Or, if you would like to make your own, I've included a few recipes at the end of this section.

Ice cubes: About 3–4 cubes for 1 serving. If you are sensitive to cold drinks, use less ice and a bit more liquid.

Fruit: Use organic fresh or frozen fruit, about 1 cup. I keep bags of frozen organic blueberries, strawberries, raspberries, cherries, mango chunks, pineapple pieces, and peach slices in my freezer. I also cut up and freeze organic bananas, which improve the texture of and add sweetness to any smoothie recipe. Of course, you can mix the fruits to make your own particular blend. If the fruit is very hard frozen, rinsing it under warm water makes it easier to blend.

Good fats: Choose one of the following:

1 tablespoon coconut oil (has a very definite taste, so try it first)
1 tablespoon flaxseed oil
2 tablespoons nut butter, such as almond butter
¼ avocado
½ cup nut milk

Protein: 1 serving vanilla or plain whey protein powder. I use whey, but you can also use rice protein or bee pollen (it is expensive).

NUT MILK RECIPE

If you would like to make your own nut milk, try this recipe.

1 cup raw nuts (brazil nuts, almonds)
3 cups filtered water

Place ingredients into a blender and blend till smooth. Strain milk and refrigerate. Use within 3 days.

(There is no added sweetener since sweetener is added to the smoothie recipe.)

QUICKIE NUT MILK

If you need nut milk right now, try this version.

2 tablespoons raw almond butter or sesame paste (tahini)
1 cup filtered water

Blend these ingredients or add them directly to your other smoothie ingredients if you are not using a nut milk as your liquid.

Lunch and Dinner

As Frank discussed in Daily Beat 7, changing your rhythm of eating to make lunch your biggest meal is one of the keys to healing Spent. Most of us are not home during the day, so making a big lunch is often not a viable option. But Frank and I have worked out a system where we make our evening meals big enough that we always have leftovers. Then we can either incorporate a piece of chicken or fish into a salad to take to work or have enough extra soup to throw into a couple of storage containers that we can just heat on the fly when we are hungry. If taking a lunch to work is not an option, just use these recipes as inspiration for what to order or buy. As you will see, all of the recipes in this section are also delicious options for dinner—just have a smaller portion.

As I said earlier, for the salads, wraps, and stir-fries my philosophy is, prepare the vegetables once but use them in many different ways.

GREEN SALADS

You can put everything, and the more things the better, into a salad, as into a conversation; but everything depends on the skill of mixing.
—Charles Dudley Warner

Many of the salad recipes include nuts, which are always optional. They can be used raw or lightly roasted, which I like as it really brings out the crunch.

ARUGULA OR MIXED BABY GREENS SALAD   *serves 2*

4 cups arugula or mixed baby greens, washed and dried
1 avocado, peeled and sliced
10 spears asparagus, steamed
2 scallions, chopped
2 tablespoons pomegranate seeds
2 hard-boiled eggs, thinly sliced

Combine all ingredients and drizzle with your favorite salad dressing.

BABY GREENS AND ROASTED BUTTERNUT SQUASH SALAD   *serves 2*

4 cups baby greens, washed and dried
1 cup of roasted butternut squash cubes (see page 297 on how to roast vegetables)
2 ounces goat cheese, crumbled
A handful of toasted pumpkin seeds

In a large salad bowl, gently mix the baby greens and roasted butternut squash cubes. Sprinkle with crumbled goat cheese and pumpkin seeds.

Drizzle with your favorite salad dressing.

SPINACH AND STRAWBERRY SALAD   *serves 2*

4 cups baby spinach leaves, washed and dried
1 pint strawberries, washed and thinly sliced
1 small red onion, thinly sliced
$\frac{1}{4}$ cup walnuts, chopped
2 ounces goat cheese

Combine all ingredients and drizzle with your favorite salad dressing.

MIXED GREENS WITH CLEMENTINES   *serves 2*

2 cups baby spinach leaves, washed and dried
1 cup arugula, washed and dried
1 small radicchio, leaves washed and coarsely shredded
1 small red onion, thinly sliced
2 clementines, peeled and sectioned
sesame seeds to sprinkle
1 mango, peeled and cut into cubes (optional)
1 avocado, peeled and cut into cubes

Combine all ingredients and drizzle with your favorite salad dressing.

SPINACH AND MUSHROOM SALAD   *serves 2*

4 cups baby spinach leaves (or any salad greens of your choice)
1 avocado, peeled and sliced
1 cup button mushrooms, cleaned and thinly sliced
2 tomatoes, sliced
$\frac{1}{2}$ cup walnuts, chopped

Combine all ingredients and drizzle with your favorite salad dressing.

WATERCRESS AND RADICCHIO SALAD   *serves 2–3*

This salad is particularly good with lemon vinaigrette.

1 large head radicchio, leaves separated, washed, dried, and
   coarsely shredded
2 cups watercress, washed and dried
15-ounce can chickpeas, drained and rinsed
½ cup walnuts, chopped

Combine all ingredients.

FENNEL AND POMEGRANATE SALAD   *serves 3–4*

4 fennel bulbs, trimmed, rinsed, and tough outer pieces removed
2 bunches of arugula or salad greens, washed and dried
Seeds from 1 pomegranate (you can substitute 2 peeled oranges
   sliced in rounds)
Handful of toasted walnuts
5 ounces goat cheese, cut into small disks (optional)

Cut fennel bulbs in half and slice thinly. Mix with arugula. Sprinkle
with pomegranate seeds and walnuts. Arrange disks of goat cheese on
top of salad and drizzle with your favorite salad dressing.

For more salad recipes, like a Chopped Romaine Salad, and an extensive list of ingredients and combinations that will allow you to create
some wonderful salads, go to www.spentmd.com. As with the
smoothie recipes, I encourage you to explore and play on your own.

GRAIN SALADS

Grains such as brown rice and quinoa can also be cooked ahead of time
and stored in the fridge till ready to use. All grain salads should be served at
room temperature.

QUINOA TABOULI SALAD *serves 4*

This is nice with lemon vinaigrette.

1 cup quinoa cooked according to package instructions—
  allow to cool
1 cup chopped tomatoes
1 cup chopped cucumbers
½ cup chopped parsley
½ cup chopped mint

Combine all ingredients in a large bowl.

QUINOA AND BLACK BEAN SALAD *serves 4*

2 teaspoons grated lime zest
2 tablespoons fresh lime juice
½ teaspoon agave
2 tablespoons extra-virgin olive oil
1 clove crushed garlic
¼ tsp ground cumin
Dash of red pepper flakes (optional)
1 cup quinoa
1 14-ounce can of organic black beans, rinsed and drained
2 tomatoes, chopped
4 scallions, chopped
¼ cup fresh cilantro, chopped
Salt and fresh-ground pepper

Mix together the lime zest, lime juice, agave, cumin, crushed garlic,
olive oil, and red pepper flakes if using them. Cook the quinoa according to instructions on the box and allow to cool. Mix all the ingredients together in a large bowl. Add salt and pepper to taste.

QUINOA WITH BUTTERNUT
SQUASH AND PINE NUTS   *serves 4*

1 large butternut squash, peeled and cut into small cubes
Extra-virgin olive oil (enough to coat butternut squash cubes
  plus 1 extra tablespoon)
Coarse sea salt
Paprika
1 large onion, chopped
1 cup quinoa, cooked according to package instructions and
  allowed to cool (or use 2 cups of leftovers)
½ cup pine nuts, lightly toasted
Chopped parsley (optional)

Preheat oven to 350 degrees. Coat the butternut squash with the olive oil and sprinkle with sea salt and paprika. Roast in oven for about 45 minutes or until lightly browned. Sauté onion in 1 tablespoon extra-virgin olive oil. Add cooked quinoa (must be cool or cold). Sauté a few minutes till heated through. Add roasted butternut squash and sprinkle with pine nuts and parsley (if desired). Remove from stove and gently mix all the ingredients together in a large bowl.

JEWELED BROWN RICE PILAF   *serves 2–3*

1 onion, diced
1 tablespoon extra-virgin olive oil
⅓ cup shredded unsweetened coconut
1 cup short-grain brown rice, cooked according to package
  instructions and allowed to cool, or use 2 cups leftover rice
½ cup lightly toasted chopped nuts (almonds, walnuts, pine
  nuts—you choose)
⅓ cup dried cranberries
Salt to taste

Sauté onion in olive oil. When opaque and starting to brown slightly, add coconut, stirring all the time. Do not let the coconut get too brown. Add cooked cold rice and cranberries and sauté for a few minutes, until heated through. Remove from stove, then sprinkle with toasted nuts and season lightly with salt.

For more salads made with grains, such as Mediterranean Brown Rice, go to www.spentmd.com.

SALAD DRESSINGS

I usually make a couple of these at a time and keep them in our fridge. Most last for five days in a well-sealed container. Another easy option is simply to drizzle a high-quality balsamic vinegar and extra-virgin olive oil directly onto your salad.

BALSAMIC VINAIGRETTE   *makes about a cup*

$\frac{2}{3}$ cup extra-virgin olive oil
$\frac{1}{3}$ cup balsamic vinegar
1 clove garlic, crushed
1 teaspoon Dijon mustard
1 teaspoon agave syrup
Pinch of salt

Combine all the ingredients in a glass jar and shake well until thoroughly blended. Adjust to taste—if it is too sharp, add a little more olive oil. (Note: Red or white wine vinegar can be substituted for the balsamic.)

LEMON VINAIGRETTE   *makes about a cup*

$\frac{3}{4}$ cup extra-virgin olive oil
$\frac{1}{4}$ cup freshly squeezed lemon juice
1 clove garlic, crushed
1 teaspoon salt
1 teaspoon mustard or to taste
Fresh ground black pepper to taste

(continued on next page)

Put all ingredients into a glass jar and shake well until thoroughly blended.

SOY VINAIGRETTE *makes about a cup*

1 tablespoon wheat-free soy sauce or tamari
$\frac{1}{2}$ cup extra-virgin olive oil
$\frac{1}{4}$ cup apple cider vinegar or juice of 2 limes
2 teaspoons agave syrup
1 small red chili, deseeded and finely chopped, or dash of red
   pepper flakes
1 tablespoon sesame oil

Put all ingredients into a glass jar and shake well until thoroughly blended.

WRAPS

Sometimes when you really want to feel your food, wraps are the answer. Wraps extend the salad concept of using your already sliced and diced ingredients and are a great way to have a salad when you are on the run. You can fill them with practically anything.

Here are two wraps just to give you a sense of what a wrap is. Really, anything is possible.

TANDOORI CHICKEN WRAP

This is based on using leftover tandoori chicken. No additional cooking is required. Fill Boston lettuce leaves (or any soft leaf lettuce) with the following:

Sliced cold cooked tandoori chicken breasts (page 295)
Tomato slices
Cucumber slices
Baby spinach leaves

Drizzle with thick Greek-style yogurt mixed with chopped fresh mint.
Wrap and enjoy.

BEEF LETTUCE WRAP

Thinly sliced leftover grilled steak
Thinly cut slices of cucumber
Carrots, cut in julienne strips
Scallions, chopped
Thin slices of radish
Thin slices of avocado
Fresh mint
Fresh cilantro
Lime juice
Extra-virgin olive oil
Salt to taste

Mix together and spoon onto soft lettuce leaves. Wrap and enjoy.

MAKE YOUR OWN WRAP

As you can see, wraps are open to interpretation. All you need to
do is use the leaves of soft lettuce (such as Boston or butter).
Rinse and dry the lettuce leaves. Lettuce leaves may be wrapped
in a damp towel and kept in fridge until ready to use. When
ready to use, place 2 tablespoons of filling on a lettuce leaf and
drizzle lightly with salad dressing. Then fold.

FILLINGS

Protein
Sliced cooked chicken breast or turkey breast (leftovers are great)
Flaked, cooked wild salmon
Thin slices of grilled grass-fed steak or lamb
Chopped or sliced hard-boiled egg

Crunch

Shredded carrots

Finely chopped celery

Finely chopped cucumber

Shredded or thinly sliced daikon radish

Shredded jicama

Greens

Arugula

Baby spinach

Flavor

Fresh mint

Fresh cilantro

For more wrap suggestions, go to www.spentmd.com.

STIR-FRIES

Stir it up.

—Bob Marley

Stir-fries are an extension of the salad bar/wrap concept since the vegetables are prepared ahead of time and stored until you are ready to use them. With the addition of protein such as fish, shrimp, organic free-range chicken, grass-fed beef or lamb, and tempeh, dinner is tasty, fast, and nutritious.

Stir-fries are light, easy to prepare, and fast to cook. The method lends itself to many different kinds of vegetables and proteins and is also a great way to use cold leftover brown rice.

Although traditionally a wok is used to stir-fry, a large skillet (frying pan) is fine too. There are a couple of basic techniques to bear in mind when making a stir-fry:

1. Have all the ingredients you will use already sliced, diced, or shredded. The harder vegetables, like onions, broccoli, carrots, and asparagus, should be the first vegetable ingredients that go into your pan, as they take a little longer to cook.

2. Have some vegetable stock on hand. I recommend prepacked organic vegetable stock (such as the Pacific brand or Trader Joe's).

3. First, heat the oil in either a wok or a large skillet over high heat. Toss a clove of garlic into the oil, and when it starts to brown, the oil is ready.

4. If you are using sliced chicken or other meat, add this next. Stir it around the pan as it cooks. Cook in small batches to avoid stewing. This should not take long. Test for doneness after a few minutes. Remove from pan and set aside.

5. Then add the spices, such as garlic, ginger, and red pepper flakes, and stir them around as they cook. It may be necessary to add a little more oil if you have stir-fried chicken or other meat first. This should take about about a minute or less.

6. Add vegetables, stir-fry for a few minutes, then add a little stock and other liquids such as soy sauce and allow all to cook until just tender. When the vegetables are almost cooked, add the cooked chicken or other meat if using.

7. Sometimes the sauce may need to be thickened. If so, when the vegetables are done, dissolve a little arrowroot in cold water and add it, stirring until the thickened sauce coats the vegetables.

8. Finally, add the final seasonings such as cilantro, toasted nuts, etc.

Now for a few recipes to get you going.

SPICY SPINACH AND MUSHROOMS serves 3–4

$\frac{1}{2}$ tablespoon olive oil
1 medium onion, chopped
1 clove garlic, crushed
1 teaspoon freshly grated ginger
1 teaspoon chili powder
$\frac{1}{2}$ pound mushrooms, thinly sliced
Salt to taste

(continued on next page)

1 pound spinach, washed, dried, and cut into ribbons (or bagged organic baby spinach)

Heat the oil in a large skillet. Add onion and garlic and stir-fry till browned. Add the spices and stir fry for about 1 minute. Add mushrooms and salt. When the mushrooms have softened, add the spinach and cook until the spinach has wilted.

STIR-FRIED GREENS   *serves 4*

2 tablespoons extra-virgin olive oil
2 cloves garlic, crushed
1 tablespoon freshly grated ginger
4 ounces baby spinach
4 ounces Swiss chard, sliced in thick ribbons
4 ounces baby bok choy, roughly chopped
4 ounces Chinese cabbage, roughly chopped
4 ounces sugar snap peas
4 tablespoons soy sauce
2 tablespoons mirin
Dash of red pepper flakes (optional)
1 tablespoon sesame seeds (optional)

Heat the oil in a large frying pan. Stir-fry the garlic and ginger briefly, 1–2 minutes. Add the vegetables in batches. Add the soy sauce and mirin. Add a dash of red pepper flakes if using. Stir-fry until the vegetables are just tender. Garnish with sesame seeds.

SAUTÉD SHRIMP WITH GARLIC AND HERBS   *serves 4*

2 tablespoons extra-virgin olive oil plus 1 tablespoon for sautéing
Juice of 1 lemon
2 cloves garlic, crushed
2 teaspoons finely chopped flat-leaf parsley
$\frac{1}{2}$ teaspoon ground thyme
$\frac{1}{2}$ teaspoon dried oregano

1 teaspoon salt

1½ pounds large peeled and deveined shrimps (heads off,
  tail on)

Dash of red pepper flakes

Lemon slices

Mix all the ingredients except the shrimp. Rinse and drain the shrimp, blotting them dry with a paper towel. Pour the marinade over and set aside for 30 minutes. Heat 1 tablespoon extra-virgin olive oil in a large pan. Add the shrimp and cook through until they have curled and turned pink. Sprinkle with red pepper flakes. Serve with lemon slices.

STIR-FRIED CHICKEN AND VEGETABLES   *serves 4–6*

You may substitute shrimp, beef, or tempeh for the chicken.

4 boneless, skinless chicken breasts, thinly sliced

4 tablespoons soy sauce

1 tablespoon mirin

2 teaspoons arrowroot

1 cup organic chicken stock (or vegetable stock if making
  vegetarian version)

3 tablespoons extra-virgin olive oil

1 large onion, sliced

2 cloves of garlic, crushed

1 tablespoon (about a 1-inch piece) ginger, grated

Dash of red pepper flakes for added kick (optional)

3 carrots, sliced in rounds

3 stalks of celery, sliced diagonally

2 cups broccoli florets

1 cup mushrooms, sliced

1 red pepper, seeds removed and sliced into thin strips

Marinate the chicken in 2 tablespoons soy sauce and mirin for 30 minutes, then drain. Mix the arrowroot, 2 tablespoons soy sauce, and

(continued on next page)

stock, set aside (thickens the sauce). Heat 1 tablespoon olive oil in a large skillet and stir-fry the chicken in batches until cooked through. Remove from pan and set aside. Wipe out the pan and heat the remaining 2 tablespoons of olive oil. When the oil is hot, add the onions, garlic, ginger, and red pepper flakes if using them. Stir-fry about 2 minutes. Add carrots, celery, and broccoli and stir-fry till almost tender. Add the mushrooms and peppers and stir-fry for 2–3 minutes. Return chicken to pan and add the thickening sauce. Cook a few more minutes, until sauce thickens. Serve with brown rice.

For more recipes and to learn how to make your own stir-fry, go to www.spentmd.com.

SOUPS

Tinned soups, unless you happen to like the taste of tin,
are universally displeasing.
—Elizabeth David, *French Country Cooking,* 1951

In the wintertime especially, soups are a big feature in our eating life. They are hearty and warming and feel nurturing. Soups do take some time to cook, so our Spent strategy is to make them on the weekend, when there is usually more time, and enjoy them during the week. I also use many of the same ingredients that we use in stir-fries or salads; in that way our strategy of preparing in advance is an added bonus. A simple soup is a great way to start a meal. A more substantial soup and salad can be a wonderful, complete meal. All of our recipes leave room for interpretation. Add and subtract as you feel inclined or lack in your pantry. *Note:* For all pureed soups I use a hand blender.

CARROT AND CORIANDER SOUP   *serves 4–6*

2 tablespoons extra-virgin olive oil
1 onion, chopped
2 cloves garlic, crushed
1 teaspoon ground thyme

2 teaspoons ground coriander

6 very large carrots (or about 8 medium carrots), peeled and
  chopped—about 3 cups

$\frac{1}{4}$ cup fresh parsley, chopped

Salt and pepper to taste

4 cups vegetable stock

Bunch of fresh cilantro, chopped

Heat the oil in a large pot, then add the onion, garlic, thyme, and coriander and sauté until soft. Add the carrots, parsley, and salt and stir-fry
for 2–3 minutes. Pour in the vegetable stock, bring to the boil, then
cover the pot and simmer for about 45 minutes, until the carrots are
tender. Remove from heat and allow to cool, then puree till smooth. If
the consistency is too thick, add more vegetable stock and puree. Adjust seasonings to taste and heat through before serving. Sprinkle with
cilantro and serve.

QUICK LENTIL AND VEGETABLE SOUP   serves 6

3 tablespoons extra-virgin olive oil

1 large onion, chopped

2 cloves fresh garlic, crushed

$\frac{1}{2}$ teaspoon ground thyme

2 large carrots, shredded (approximately 2 cups)

1 cup red lentils, rinsed

6 cups vegetable stock

1 bay leaf

$\frac{1}{2}$ cup parsley, chopped

2 cups cabbage, shredded

1 tablespoon tomato paste

1 teaspoon salt

Freshly ground pepper

Heat the oil in a large pot and add the onion, garlic, thyme, and carrots. Stir-fry for a few minutes and then add remaining ingredients.
Bring to the boil, cover the pot, and simmer for about 30 minutes,

(continued on next page)

stirring occasionally. For the best flavor, allow to cool, then reheat before serving. Check seasonings before serving and remove the bay leaf.

This soup tends to thicken, so add more vegetable stock if necessary.

BUTTERNUT SQUASH AND
ROOT VEGETABLE SOUP *serves 8*

3 tablespoons olive oil
1 large onion, peeled and chopped
2 cloves fresh garlic, crushed
1 large butternut squash, peeled, seeded, and cubed
3 carrots, peeled and chopped
3 parsnips, peeled and chopped
1 sweet potato, peeled and chopped
2 leeks, cleaned and chopped (white parts only)
1 teaspoon ground thyme
Salt and freshly ground pepper to taste
8 cups vegetable stock

Heat the oil in a large pot, add the onion and garlic, and stir-fry till the onion is soft. Add the remaining vegetables, thyme, salt, and pepper and stir-fry for a few minutes. Pour in the stock and bring to the boil. Reduce heat, cover, and simmer till all the vegetables are soft (about 45 minutes). Cool, then puree. Adjust seasonings and reheat before serving.

SIMPLE BROCCOLI SOUP *serves 6–8*

This soup can be a blueprint for many simple vegetable soups. Try it with cauliflower or a mixture of squashes. Play with the herbs and spices.

1 tablespoon olive oil
1 medium onion, chopped
2 cloves fresh garlic, crushed
2 pounds fresh broccoli, rinsed and chopped

1 teaspoon ground thyme
Salt and freshly ground pepper to taste
6–8 cups vegetable stock (depending on how thick you want
the soup)
Fresh chopped parsley, chives, or dill

In a large pot, heat the oil and sauté the onion and garlic till onion is soft and translucent. Add the remaining ingredients and bring to the boil. Cover, reduce heat, and simmer till the broccoli is tender, about 40 minutes. Check seasoning. Puree the soup and garnish with fresh parsley, chives, or dill.

For more soup recipes, including my favorite vegetable soup, go to www.spentmd.com.

COMFORT MEALS

Sometimes soups, stir-fries, salads, and wraps just aren't enough, particularly in the winter, when we want something warm and perhaps a bit more substantial. At our house, when we are feeling like this in the summer, it means grilling some fish, chicken, or meat and vegetables outside. In the winter, it means roasting vegetables and broiling some fish, chicken, or meat. (Pan-frying, sautéing, stir-frying, grilling, and broiling fish, chicken, and meat are *all* healthy cooking options.) Occasionally, we'll have brown rice pasta with sautéed or roasted vegetables or a spicy tomato sauce.

More often than not, when I cook chicken, fish, or meat, I use a rub or a marinade. Spice rubs keep for up to 6 months in a cool, dry place, and the marinades keep for a week in the fridge. This really simplifies preparing the protein portion of the meal. If I feel like something spicy, I use the "spicy" rub; if something more "herby," then perhaps the olive oil, garlic, and herb marinade. There are so many options that our taste buds are always happy and our bodies are grateful for being well fed. *Note:* I always date the containers so that I know how long they've been around.

Rubs and marinades are a great way to impart flavor to food. Rubs are made of dried herbs, spices, salt, and pepper. The dry mix is rubbed onto the food with your fingers till it is lightly coated, or you can put the food in a plastic bag, add the rub mix, and shake the bag till the food is coated.

(This way is useful if both sides of the food need to be coated.) The food either can be cooked right away or can sit for a few hours covered in the fridge till you are ready to make it. Because dry rubs can be made in advance, you can double or triple the quantities. You will need about 1½–2 teaspoons of a dry rub for every pound of meat, fish, or chicken and a little more if you use the bag method.

Marinades are similar to rubs except that they are liquid—olive oil, lemon juice, vinegar, and soy sauce in any combination are part of the mix, and the food is soaked in the marinade for a couple of hours or overnight. However, fish should not marinate overnight as it tends to make the fish mushy. Don't worry about making too much, as any unused marinade can be stored in the fridge for up to 1 week.

Preparing poultry, meat, and fish with rubs and marinades is easy and delicious.

RUBS

Note: Even though I have specified that some of the following rub and marinade recipes are for certain foods, they can also be used on chicken, lamb, or fish.

ALL-PURPOSE RUB   *about 3 tablespoons*

1 teaspoon garlic powder
1 teaspoon ground thyme
3 teaspoons dried rosemary
3 teaspoons dried oregano
1 teaspoon salt
1 teaspoon freshly ground black pepper

Blend together and rub on well until meat is evenly coated. Pan-fry the meat on grill pan or skillet, broil, or roast in oven.

CAJUN RUB   *about 10 tablespoons*

3 tablespoons chili powder
2 tablespoons paprika

2 tablespoons coarse salt
1 teaspoon garlic powder
2 teaspoons ground cumin
1 teaspoon dried oregano
2 tablespoons mustard powder
½ teaspoon ground cinnamon
1 teaspoon freshly ground black pepper

Rub fish or chicken breasts with a little olive oil before applying the rub. Place the meat on a lightly oiled broiler pan and broil in the oven, turning once, until cooked. (If using fish with skin on, apply rub only to the skinless side; apply to both sides of chicken breasts.)

INDIAN SPICE RUB *about 2 tablespoons*

1 teaspoon ground cumin
1 teaspoon ground coriander
1 teaspoon ground turmeric
1 teaspoon garam masala
Pinch of cayenne pepper
½ teaspoon garlic powder
½ teaspoon ground ginger
Salt to taste

Blend together and rub on well until meat is evenly coated. (I like to rub a little lemon juice and olive oil directly onto chicken breasts before using the rub.) Grill on an oiled grill pan, broil, or roast in an oven. Serve with lemon wedges.

MARINADES

LEMON AND OLIVE OIL MARINADE *serves 4*

This recipe makes a large quantity, so use half and keep the rest to use within a week.

(continued on next page)

¾ *cup extra-virgin olive oil*

Juice of 2 lemons

1 tablespoon freshly chopped parsley

1 teaspoon salt

4 cloves garlic, crushed

1 teaspoon mustard powder

1 teaspoon dried oregano

1 teaspoon freshly ground black pepper

4 boneless and skinless chicken breasts

Combine all the ingredients and marinate the chicken breasts for at least one hour or overnight. Remove from the marinade and pan-fry in a lightly oiled grill pan or skillet until cooked through, about 4–5 minutes per side.

SPICY MARINADE

Makes about ½ cup, sufficient for 1½ pounds of meat.

¼ *cup red wine vinegar*

¼ *cup extra-virgin olive oil*

1–2 teaspoons freshly ground black pepper

1 teaspoon dried oregano

½–*1 teaspoon crushed red pepper (or* ½–*1 teaspoon cayenne) to taste*

1 clove garlic, crushed

½ *teaspoon paprika*

1 teaspoon salt

Combine ingredients and marinate food for at least one hour or overnight. Remove from marinade and pan-fry on lightly oiled grill pan or skillet.

TANDOORI MARINADE

This marinade can be used for boneless, skinless chicken breasts, lamb chops, or salmon. If using chicken, make a couple of diagonal slashes into the chicken breast before marinading.

$\frac{3}{4}$ cup plain yogurt (do not use Greek-style yogurt,
  as it's too thick)
4 cloves fresh garlic, crushed
1 teaspoon garlic powder
2 teaspoons freshly grated ginger
1 teaspoon salt
$1\frac{1}{2}$ teaspoons ground cumin
$\frac{1}{2}$ teaspoon cayenne pepper
2 teaspoons ground coriander
1 tablespoon paprika
$\frac{1}{2}$ teaspoon turmeric
$\frac{1}{2}$ teaspoon ground cinnamon
Juice of a large lemon (about 2 tablespoons)

Mix all ingredients together in a large glass bowl. Marinate meat overnight. Pour off the excess marinade (reserve for basting). Place on a lightly oiled rack in a roasting pan. Cook in the oven on the lowest shelf at 350 degrees until cooked; baste and turn halfway through cooking.

MUSTARD AND ROSEMARY MARINADE

2 tablespoons whole-grain mustard
1 tablespoon extra-virgin olive oil
Juice of 1 lemon
1 clove garlic, crushed
1 tablespoon fresh rosemary, chopped
Salt and freshly ground pepper to taste

(continued on next page)

Mix ingredients together and rub over 1½ pounds boneless, skinless chicken breasts, salmon fillets, or lamb chops (coat only the skinless side of salmon). Allow to stand for 10 minutes. Pan-fry meat on lightly oiled grill pan or skillet or broil in oven, turning once, until cooked.

VEGETABLES

To me, there is nothing more delicious than a bite of fish with a piece of grilled zucchini, a bite of sautéed chicken with a bit of sautéed spinach, or a bite of steak with a piece of roasted potato. That is what this section is about: making each bite of food more enjoyable. Allow the flavor of the rubs and marinades to expand into the vegetables on your plate.

SAUTÉED SPINACH (OR SWISS CHARD OR KALE)   *serves 4*

1 tablespoon extra-virgin olive oil
1 clove garlic, crushed
1½ pounds spinach (packaged organic baby spinach works well)
Salt and freshly ground pepper

Heat the oil in a frying pan. Add the crushed garlic and sauté briefly. Add baby spinach in handfuls so as not to overload the pan. Cook until just wilted. Add salt and freshly ground pepper to taste.

MEDLEY OF SAUTÉED MUSHROOMS   *serves 4*

3 tablespoons extra-virgin olive oil
2 cloves garlic, finely chopped
1 pound mushrooms (any variety), wiped clean and sliced thinly
½ teaspoon dried oregano
Salt and freshly ground pepper
¼ cup fresh parsley, chopped

Heat the olive oil in a large frying pan. Add garlic and sauté a few minutes. Add the mushrooms and oregano and stir until the mushrooms begin to change color, about 5 to 7 minutes. Add salt and freshly ground pepper to taste. Garnish with chopped parsley.

MAKE YOUR OWN VEGETABLES

Other than stir-frying, my favorite ways to prepare vegetables are roasting, sautéing, and steaming. For sautéing and steaming, vegetables are sliced, diced, or cubed. Leafy greens can be left whole or torn into large ribbons. Vegetables should be cut uniformly so that they cook evenly.

Steamed Vegetables

Most vegetables can be steamed except starchy ones like potatoes. Pour about 2 cups of water into a large pot, then put the vegetables into a steamer basket in the pot. (Make sure water does not come through the steamer basket.) Bring to a boil. Steam vegetables until a fork can just slide into them. Season with salt and pepper and lemon juice. A great seasoning to try is gomasio (sesame seeds and sea salt) or sea salt with sea vegetables.

Sautéed Vegetables

Sautéing vegetables is very similar to stir-frying them. The main ingredients are extra-virgin olive oil, garlic (thinly sliced or crushed), salt, and freshly ground black pepper. Fresh or dried herbs such as oregano, basil, and rosemary are optional, but add great flavor. Heat about 2 tablespoons of extra-virgin olive oil in a large skillet over medium to high heat, add garlic, vegetables, salt, and pepper and cook until the vegetables are just tender.

Roasted Vegetables

Roasting is not just for potatoes. Most vegetables, except for leafy ones, can be roasted in the oven. Just toss the vegetables with enough olive oil to coat them, sprinkle with coarse salt, and roast in a moderately hot oven (350° or 375° F.) until golden brown. Sprigs of fresh herbs are a wonderful addition. Most vegetables take about 45 minutes to an hour to roast, but some, like broccoli and asparagus, take about 20 minutes (keep checking to make sure they are not browning too quickly). Leftover roasted vegetables are great in salads.

Instead of French fries, roast thin slices of parsnips in the oven with a drizzle of olive oil to coat them and a sprinkle of coarse sea salt. Preheat the oven to 350° F.; when hot, roast parsnips on a baking sheet until tender and golden on the outside (45 minutes to 1 hour). These could not be more delicious!

ONE-DISH MEALS

For those nights when you drag your feet home—hopefully this is happening less and less—here are a few easy and comforting one-pot meals.

EASY ONE-DISH ROAST   *serves 4*

Preheat oven to 375° F. Season four bone-in, skin-on chicken breasts with salt, pepper, oregano, garlic powder, and paprika and place in an ovenproof roasting dish, or use the all-purpose rub. Arrange an assortment of peeled and sliced parsnips, carrots, sweet potatoes, butternut squash, and wedges of red onion around the chicken. Throw in three cloves of garlic, peeled and sliced. Drizzle the vegetables with a little olive oil. Roast at 375° F. until the chicken is cooked through, about 40 minutes.

ROASTED FISH FILLETS WITH FRESH HERBS   *serves 4*

4 fish fillets (6 ounces each, skin on)
Juice of 1 lemon
Salt and ground black pepper to taste
1 clove garlic, crushed
½ cup of chopped fresh herbs (parsley, dill, garlic, oregano,
  basil—pick your favorites)
Extra-virgin olive oil
Lemon wedges (optional)

Preheat the oven to 375° F. Moisten the fish with the lemon juice. Season with salt and pepper. Mix together the garlic, herbs, and a little extra-virgin olive oil to hold the herbs together. Spread the herb mix evenly on the fish fillets. Place the fillets skin side down on a lightly oiled baking sheet and roast in the oven until cooked (flake easily with a fork and are opaque), about 12–15 minutes, depending on the thickness of the fish. Serve with additional lemon wedges if desired.

VEGETABLE CURRY   *serves 4*

1 onion, chopped
2 cloves garlic, crushed
2 tablespoons extra-virgin olive oil
$\frac{1}{2}$ teaspoon curry powder
1 teaspoon cumin
$\frac{1}{2}$ teaspoon coriander
$\frac{1}{4}$ teaspoon cinnamon
$\frac{1}{4}$ teaspoon ground ginger
$\frac{1}{4}$ teaspoon tumeric
$\frac{1}{2}$ teaspoon salt
$\frac{1}{2}$ butternut squash, peeled and cut into small cubes
$\frac{3}{4}$ cup water
1 large sweet potato, peeled and cut into small cubes
$\frac{1}{2}$ head cauliflower, cut into small florets
$\frac{3}{4}$ cup frozen organic peas
$\frac{1}{2}$ teaspoon garam masala
Cilantro (optional)

Fry the onion and garlic in olive oil until the onions are soft and opaque. Add the spices and salt and saute a few minutes, until you can smell the aroma of the spices. Stir the spices from the bottom of the pot occasionally. Add the butternut squash and sauté about 10 minutes, stirring occasionally. Add 1 or 2 tablespoons of water to prevent sticking. Add sweet potato and sauté another 10 minutes, stirring occasionally. Add the rest of the water, and scrape all the spices up from the bottom of the pot. Add cauliflower and peas on top of the butternut and sweet potato; do not stir. Cook until vegetables are tender, about 10–15 minutes. Just before serving, add garam masala and stir through. Sprinkle with cilantro and serve with brown rice.

BROWN RICE PASTA WITH
GARLIC ROASTED VEGETABLES   *serves 3–4*

Any vegetables that roast well can be used.

2 large carrots, peeled and sliced into thin diagonals
2 zucchini, cut into $\frac{1}{4}$-inch diagonals
2 fennel bulbs, thinly sliced
1 red pepper, seeds removed and thinly sliced
$\frac{1}{2}$ pound green beans, sliced in half
Extra-virgin olive oil
Coarse salt and freshly ground pepper
1 tablespoon dried oregano
2–3 cloves garlic, peeled and thinly sliced
Brown rice pasta (any shape)
$\frac{1}{2}$ cup of sundried tomatoes in oil, drained

Preheat oven to 350° F. In a large bowl, toss the vegetables with enough extra-virgin olive oil to coat. Place on a large baking sheet (or two) and sprinkle lightly with coarse salt, black pepper, and oregano. Toss in the garlic. Roast in the oven until tender and slightly browned, about 40 minutes. Cook the pasta according to the package instructions and drain. Add the sundried tomatoes and roasted vegetables, garlic, and any leftover olive oil from roasting, toss gently and serve.

TOMATO SAUCE WITH OLIVES AND CAPERS   *serves 4*

This sauce works with just about everything, from brown rice pasta to a piece of fish or chicken.

2 tablespoons extra virgin olive oil
2 cloves garlic, crushed
2 cups (28-ounce can, drained) chopped-up tomatoes
Dash of red pepper flakes (optional)
$\frac{1}{2}$ cup kalamata olives, pitted
$\frac{1}{4}$ cup capers, rinsed and drained

Heat the oil, add the garlic, and cook about 1 minute (do not let the garlic get brown). Add the tomatoes and red pepper flakes if using and cook for about 8–10 minutes, stirring occasionally until tomatoes break down. Add the olives and capers. Cook for an additional minute or two, stirring frequently. Spoon sauce over grilled fish or chicken breasts; mix with cooked shrimp; or use as a sauce for brown rice pasta.

Snack Attack

Here are a few ideas and recipes for the between-meals meals.

TRAIL MIX

$\frac{1}{2}$ cup raw almonds
$\frac{1}{2}$ cup raw walnuts
$\frac{1}{2}$ cup raw cashew nuts
$\frac{1}{2}$ cup raw brazil nuts
$\frac{1}{2}$ cup raw sunflower seeds
$\frac{1}{2}$ cup raw pumpkin seeds
$\frac{1}{2}$ cup cocoa nibs
$\frac{1}{2}$ cup chopped dates
$\frac{1}{2}$ cup chopped organic apricots (unsulphered)

Mix together and keep in an airtight jar.

Portion allowed for a snack = $\frac{1}{2}$ cup

OTHER SNACKS

1 cup plain organic yogurt with ½ cup organic berries such as blueberries, raspberries, or strawberries or a mix of the berries (if you can get goat yogurt, please try it; it's delicious and easily digested)

1 cup plain organic yogurt mixed with ½ tablespoon agave syrup and ¼ cup chopped raw walnuts (again, please try goat yogurt)

¼ avocado and sliced tomato on toasted Ezekiel bread

Drained sardines in olive oil on toasted Ezekiel bread, with tomato slices

½ cup organic berries

A piece of fruit

Apple slices with 1 tablespoon of raw almond butter

Protein shake or smoothie (see page 269)

Hummus with cucumber spears, carrot sticks, and/or celery sticks

1 ounce of dark chocolate (at least 65%)

Sweets and Treats

Strength is the capacity to break a chocolate bar into four pieces with your bare hands—and then eat just one of the pieces.

—Judith Viorst

Though I know you are off sugar, here are a few treats to satisfy your sweet tooth.

CLEMENTINE SEGMENTS DIPPED IN DARK CHOCOLATE

4 clementines
16 ounces dark chocolate
¼ cup shredded coconut
¼ cup toasted chopped almonds

Peel and segment the clementines. Melt the chocolate in a double boiler. Dip the clementine segments into the melted chocolate and sprinkle with toasted chopped almonds or shredded unsweetened coconut.

PAPAYA AND MANGO SALAD

1 large papaya, halved, seeded, peeled, and cut into thin slices
1 large mango, peeled and thinly sliced
1 lime

Arrange the fruit on a large plate. Squeeze the juice of 1 lime over the fruit.

WALNUT DATE BALLS

2 cups coarsely chopped walnuts
1 cup dates, pits removed
3 tablespoons fresh lemon juice
Pinch of sea salt
$\frac{1}{3}$ cup finely shredded unsweetened coconut

Chop the nuts in a food processor. Add the dates, lemon juice, and salt. Pulse until mixture is well blended and starts to stick together. Roll into small balls and roll into shredded coconut. Place in the fridge to harden for $\frac{1}{2}$ hour before eating.

BANANA STRAWBERRY SORBET

1 banana, peeled, cut into chunks, and frozen
1 cup frozen strawberries
$\frac{1}{2}$ teaspoon vanilla extract (optional)
1 teaspoon agave syrup (optional)

In a food processor, combine all ingredients, and process until well blended, smooth, and creamy. Serve immediately or refreeze for later.

CHOCOLATE FUDGE (HALVA)

16-ounce jar of nut butter (almond, cashew, or sesame paste)
$\frac{1}{4}$ cup organic cocoa powder
$\frac{1}{2}$ cup agave syrup
2 teaspoons vanilla extract
1 teaspoon sea salt

Mix all ingredients in a food processor (the mixture will be a little crumbly, but as you pat it into the baking dish, it will become smooth). Line a baking dish with parchment paper. Spoon the mixture into the dish and pat down. Cover well with cling wrap and place in

(continued on next page)

freezer for about 1 hour. Remove from freezer and cut into small squares. Keep in the freezer to prevent fudge from turning soft and mushy.

CHOCOLATE AVOCADO SMOOTHIE   *serves 2*

1 cup coconut water (or $\frac{1}{2}$ cup nut milk and $\frac{1}{2}$ cup filtered water)
$\frac{1}{4}$ avocado
$\frac{1}{4}$ cup raw cocoa powder
1 serving or 3–4 tablespoons whey protein powder
1 tablespoon agave syrup
4 ice cubes

Blend in a blender until smooth and creamy.

For variety, add $\frac{1}{4}$ cup fresh mint leaves.

Resources

Frank Lipman, M.D.
32 West 22nd Street, 5th Floor
New York, NY 10010
Telephone 212-255-1800
Fax 212-255-0714
www.spentmd.com
Companion Web site for the book.

Institute for Functional Medicine
Telephone 800-228-0622 (toll free)
www.functionalmedicine.org
For a listing of doctors trained in functional medicine.

Food

NONPROFIT GENERAL INFORMATION ORGANIZATIONS

Food News
www.foodnews.org
*This features a great downloadable guide to the twelve fruits and veggies with the
most and least pesticides so you'll know which ones to buy organic and which conventionally grown ones are okay when organic isn't available.*

Local Harvest
www.localharvest.org

The freshest, healthiest, most flavorful organic food is what's grown closest to you. Use this Web site to find farmers' markets, family farms, and other sources of sustainably grown food in your area, where you can buy produce, grass-fed meats, and many other goodies.

Food Routes
www.foodroutes.org

The Food Routes Find Good Food map can help you connect with local farmers so that you can find the freshest, tastiest food possible. On the interactive map, you can find listings of local farmers, community supported agriculture, and markets near you.

Farmers' Markets
www.ams.usda.gov/farmersmarkets

A national listing of farmers' markets.

Community Involved in Sustaining Agriculture (CISA)
www.buylocalfood.com

CISA is dedicated to sustaining agriculture and promoting the products of small farms.

Community Supported Agriculture (CSA)
www.nal.usda.gov/afsic/csa

Community Supported Agriculture is a community of individuals who pledge to support a farm operation so that the farmland becomes, either legally or spiritually, the community's farm, with the growers and consumers providing mutual support and sharing the risks and benefits of food production. Typically, members or "shareholders" of the farm or garden pledge in advance to cover the anticipated costs of the farm's operation and farmer's salary. In return, they receive shares in the farm's bounty throughout the growing season, as well as gain satisfaction from reconnecting to the land and participating directly in food production.

Slow Food USA

www.slowfoodusa.org

Slow Food USA is a nonprofit educational organization dedicated to supporting and celebrating the food traditions of North America through programs and activities dedicated to Taste Education, Defending Biodiversity, and Building Food Communities. Slow Food USA envisions a future food system that is based on the principles of high quality and taste, environmental sustainability, and social justice. It seeks to catalyze a broad cultural shift away from the destructive effects of an industrial food system and fast life, toward the regenerative cultural, social, and economic benefits of a sustainable food system, regional food traditions, the pleasures of the table, and a slower and more harmonious rhythm of life.

Center for Food Safety

www.centerforfoodsafety.org

The Center for Food Safety provides leadership in legal, scientific, and grassroots efforts to address the increasing concerns about the impacts of our food production system on human health, animal welfare, and the environment.

Organic Consumers Association (OCA)

www.organicconsumers.org

The Organic Consumers Association (OCA) is a grassroots nonprofit public interest organization that deals with crucial issues of food safety, industrial agriculture, genetic engineering, corporate accountability, and environmental sustainability. It monitors and reports on important issues impacting all things organic: food and produce, cosmetics, personal care products, etc. It offers a daily roundup of related news from around the Web, plus several key action campaigns that give you the opportunity to contact your representatives in Washington (if you're an American citizen, anyway) and let your voice be heard.

The Organic Pages Online

www.theorganicpages.com

The Organic Pages Online is part of the Organic Trade Association (OTA), which provides a quick, easy way to find certified organic products, producers, ingredients, supplies, and services offered by OTA members, as well as items of interest to the entire organic community.

Eat Well Guide
Telephone 212-991-1858
www.eatwellguide.org

The Eat Well Guide is an online directory of sustainably raised meat, poultry, dairy, and eggs from farms, stores, restaurants, inns, hotels, and online outlets in the United States and Canada. You can simply enter your zip or postal code to find local products that were raised sustainably, including no antibiotics, no added hormones, pasture-raised, grass-fed, and organic. New listings are being added on a continual basis.

Weston A. Price Foundation
www.westonaprice.org

The goal of the Weston A. Price Foundation is to restore nutrient-dense traditional foods to the human diet through education, research, and activism. In order to achieve its goal, the foundation supports accurate nutrition instruction, organic and biodynamic farming, pasture feeding of livestock, and community-supported farms.

Citizens for Health
www.citizens.org

Citizens for Health is a national grassroots advocacy organization committed to protecting and expanding your natural health choices.

ORGANIC PRODUCTS IN GENERAL

ShopNatural
Telephone 520-884-0745
www.shopnatural.com

ShopNatural is the online division of the ShopNatural Cooperative, which is operated as a cooperative and has been in business in Tucson, Arizona, since 1974. It is owned by its members, who participate in purchasing products and providing input and feedback on the products and services the company should carry. They carry more than six thousand products.

Organic Provisions
Telephone 800-490-0044 (toll free)
www.orgfood.com

Organic Provisions is a convenient way of ordering a wide array of quality natural foods and products from your home. More than two thousand healthy items, including hard-to-find products, are available by mail order.

Organic Planet
Telephone 415-765-5590
www.organic-planet.com

Organic Planet provides reasonably priced, high-quality organic foods and friendly service.

Diamond Organics
Telephone 888-674-2642 (toll free)
www.diamondorganics.com

Diamond Organics provides organically grown food and other organic products by direct home delivery. From California, it provides a consistent year-round selection of organically grown fresh fruits and vegetables with next-day air delivery.

Earthbound Farm
Telephone 800-690-3200 (toll free)
www.earthboundfarm.com

Packaged organic produce that will make having a salad bar in your fridge easy.

GRASS-FED MEATS, POULTRY, EGGS

Eatwild.com
Telephone 866-453-8489 (toll free, United States only)
Telephone 253-759-2318 (from outside United States)
www.eatwild.com

Eatwild.com is a great source for safe, healthy, natural, and nutritious grass-fed beef, lamb, goat, bison, poultry, pork, and dairy products. To find a local farmer, go to its directory of farmers.

Grassland Beef
Telephone 877-383-0051 (toll free)
www.uswellnessmeats.com
The mission of Grassland Beef is to provide superior-quality, grass-fed beef as part of its overall goal of improving family nutrition, rural communities, and the environment.

FISH

Vital Choice
Telephone 866-482-5887 (toll free)
www.vitalchoice.com
Fresh-caught, sustainably harvested Alaskan salmon and other Alaskan and northwest Pacific seafood delivered right to your door.

GLUTEN-FREE RESOURCES

Glutenfree.com
Telephone 800-291-8386 (toll free)
www.glutenfree.com

Glutino
Telephone 800-363-3438 (toll free)
www.glutino.com

Gillian's Foods
Telephone 781-586-0086
www.gilliansfoods.com

Gluten Solutions
Telephone 888-845-8836 (toll free)
www.glutensolutions.com

The Really Great Food Company
Telephone 800-593-5377 (toll free)
www.reallygreatfood.com

Cream Hill Estates
Telephone 866-727-3628 (toll free)
www.creamhillestates.com

Gluten Free Oats
Telephone 307-754-2058
www.glutenfreeoats.com

COCONUT PRODUCTS

Wilderness Family Naturals
www.wildernessfamilynaturals.com

Amazon.com
www.amazon.com
Zico coconut water and other brands are available here.

Toxicity and the Environment

NONPROFITS

Environmental Working Group
www.ewg.org
As the name reveals, this organization focuses on the environment, educating read-ers with articles about toxic chemicals in foods and consumer products, threats to the environment, and corruption between commercial interests and government regula-tors.

The Collaborative on Health and the Environment
www.cheforhealth.org
The Collaborative on Health and the Environment is a nonpartisan partnership network working to further knowledge, action, and cooperation regarding environ-mental contributors to disease.

Center for Children's Health and the Environment
www.childenvironment.org

The Center for Children's Health and the Environment (CCHE) at Mount Sinai Hospital is the nation's first academic research and policy center to examine the links between exposure to toxic pollutants and childhood illness.

Healthy Child Healthy World
www.healthychild.org

Healthy Child Healthy World is a national nonprofit organization dedicated to educating the public, specifically parents and caregivers, about environmental toxins that affect children's health.

Healthy Toys
www.healthytoys.org

Healthy Toys.org was launched to address the failures of our current system to regulate chemicals in products, as no government agency is adequately ensuring that children's products do not contain harmful chemicals. Nor does any agency require labeling or disclosure to inform consumers about the chemical components of children's products. Healthy Toys.org is a first step in providing parents, grandparents, and others who care about children with the information they need to make better choices when purchasing toys and other children's products.

Coming Clean
www.come-clean.org

Coming Clean is a network of groups and individuals whose common goal is to work together on chemical policies and campaigns to protect the public and the environment from exposure to harmful and unstudied chemicals. Coming Clean serves as an incubator for these campaigns and strategies and has another Web site dedicated to body burden: www.chemicalbodyburden.org.

SweetPoison.com
www.sweetpoison.com

Information on aspartame and Splenda.

Home Products

Green Home
Telephone 877-282-6400 (toll free)
www.greenhome.com

An online department store and resource for all your green living needs; a place to find up-to-date, credible information to help you make decisions about how to improve the quality of your life.

Gaiam
Telephone 877-989-6321 (toll free)
www.gaiam.com

Gaiam is a provider of information, goods, and services to customers who value the environment, a sustainable economy, healthy lifestyles, alternative health care, and personal development.

H3Environmental Corporation
Telephone 818-766-1787
www.h3environmental.com

The "H3" in H3Environmental refers to the three homes we inhabit: the home within ourselves, the literal home we live in, and our home on the planet. It provides healthy, sophisticated, elegant home products as well as valuable and practical healthy home education and information.

EcoChoices Natural Living Store
Telephone 626-969-3707
www.ecochoices.com

Environmentally friendly products for the home.

Allergy Buyers Club
Telephone 888-236-7231 (toll free)
www.allergybuyersclub.com

Specializes in allergy relief products and education on the control and prevention of allergies, sinusitis, and asthma. Its best-in-class products are natural, green, and hypoallergenic, perfect for a clean, healthy home that is free of pollutants.

Lifekind
Telephone 800-284-4983 (toll free)
www.lifekind.com

Lifekind provides the information and products to help reduce your daily exposure to hazardous chemicals. It offers certified organic and safer alternatives to products made with unhealthy and toxic ingredients.

WATER FILTERS

Custom Pure
Telephone 206-363-0039
www.custompure.com/doc/water.htm

Custom Pure offers a variety of filtration systems to meet your particular needs. But even more important, its trained professionals can help you select the right equipment, install it properly, and maintain it for optimum performance. From drinking water to shower water to small industrial applications, Custom Pure can help with information and products.

AIR FILTERS

AllerAir
Telephone 888-852-8247 (toll free)
www.allerair.com

AllerAir is dedicated to offering you the safest, most effective air-cleaning technology available. It has a wide selection in many styles and sizes, having developed more than a hundred models to meet any air purification need.

NONTOXIC HOUSEHOLD CLEANING PRODUCTS

Seventh Generation
www.seventhgeneration.com

Ecover
www.ecover.com

Dr. Bronner's Magic Soaps
www.drbronner.com

Life Without Plastic
www.lifewithoutplastic.com
LWP is an Internet-based retailer and distributor offering customers around the world nonplastic alternatives for day-to-day products such as water bottles, food storage containers, and children's dishes, bottles, and cups. Also has some important basic facts on plastics.

Cosmetics

NONPROFITS

Cosmetic Safety Database
www.cosmeticdatabase.com
Check out the safety of your skin care products. The Environmental Working Group's (EWG's) six-month investigation into the health and safety assessments of more than 10,000 personal care product ingredients found major gaps in the regulatory safety net for these products.

The Campaign for Safe Cosmetics
www.safecosmetics.org
The Campaign for Safe Cosmetics is a coalition of public health, educational, religious, labor, women's, environmental, and consumer groups. Its goal is to protect the health of consumers and workers by requiring the health and beauty industry to phase out the use of chemicals that are known or suspected carcinogens, mutagens, and reproductive toxins.

NATURAL COSMETICS

Dr. Hauschka Skin Care
www.drhauschka.com

Sophyto Organics
www.sophytoorganics.com

Avalon Organics
www.avalonorganics.com

Evan Healy Skincare
www.evanhealy.com

Sumbody Skincare
www.sumbody.com

Supplements

ConsumerLab.com
www.consumerlab.com
ConsumerLab.com ("CL") provides independent test results and information to help consumers and health care professionals evaluate health, wellness, and nutrition products. It publishes results of its tests online, including listings of brands that have passed its testing.

Yoga Supplies

Tools for Yoga
Telephone 888-678-YOGA (toll-free)
www.toolsforyoga.net

Gaiam
Telephone 877-989-6321 (toll-free)
www.gaiam.com

Yoga Accessories
www.yogaaccessories.com

Yoga Props
www.yogaprops.com

Hugger Mugger Yoga Products
www.huggermugger.com

Exercise

Power Systems
www.power-systems.com
Web site to buy exercise equipment; articles on fitness and exercise as well.

Exertools
www.exertools.com

Movement

Gabrielle Roth
www.gabrielleroth.com

Kristi Anderson
www.posturerx.com

Light Therapy

Center for Environmental Therapeutics
www.cet.org
*The Center for Environmental Therapeutics is an independent, nonprofit profes-
sional agency offering authoritative information on nonmedication treatments for
seasonal affective disorder, nonseasonal depression, and circadian rhythm sleep disorders.*

LIGHT BOXES

The SunBox Company
www.sunbox.com

BioBrite
www.biobrite.com

VITAMIN D RESOURCES

Information on vitamin D
www.vitamindcouncil.org

Music for Brain Wave Entrainment

The Monroe Institute
Telephone 866-881-3440 (toll free)
www.monroeinstitute.org

Healing Sounds
Telephone 800-246-9764 (toll free)
www.healingsounds.com

Get Involved

Global Volunteers
www.globalvolunteers.org
Global Volunteers recruits, trains, and puts volunteers to work and has been doing so since 1984. Volunteers pay upward of $2,000 for longer programs, but discounts are available for those who go with a friend or are students. The variety of programs around the world means there's likely to be a program that appeals to your particular interests or skills.

i-to-i
www.i-to-i.com
The volunteer travel organization i-to-i sends thousands of people to important projects around the world each year. It offers about 500 volunteer projects in more than twenty different countries. Volunteers work on community development, conservation, teaching, building, media, health care, and sports-coaching projects.

Airline Ambassadors International
www.airlineamb.org
Airline Ambassadors International is a group founded by an American Airlines flight attendant and staffed by volunteer airline flight attendants, pilots, and regular travelers. Airline Ambassadors International runs about six to eight special missions each month, and participants pay their basic costs. But it's the value here that really counts—what you give, and give back, to people who really need the help.

Transitions Abroad
www.transitionsabroad.com
A great resource for studying, working, volunteering, and living abroad.

The Cultural Explorer
www.theculturalexplorer.com
If you are looking for a cultural or philanthropic travel experience in South Africa, the Cultural Explorer will give you the opportunity to make a real difference as you travel and contribute to the people and communities you visit.

Functional Testing Laboratories

Genova Diagnostics
www.gdx.net
Previously known as Great Smokies Diagnostic Laboratory.

Metametrix Clinical Laboratory
Telephone 800-221-4640 (toll-free)
www.metametrix.com

Doctor's Data
Telephone 800-323-2784 (toll free)
www.doctorsdata.com

NOTES

Spent: An Epidemic of Exhaustion

1. Sidney MacDonald Baker with Karen Baar, *The Circadian Prescription: Get in Step with Your Body's Natural Rhythms to Maximize Energy, Vitality, and Longevity* (New York: Putnam, 2000), pp. 17–25.
2. J. S. Takahashi and M. Zatz, "Regulation of Circadian Rhythmicity," *Science* 217, no. 4565 (1982): 1104–1111.
3. Harvard Medical School press release, "Researchers Discover Mechanism That Drives Daily Body Rhythms," January 14, 1999, available at www.sciencedaily.com/releases/1999/01/990114075249.

Prepare

1. Forbes.com source: IMS Health, a health care information company. Twelve Months Ending December 2005.
2. Michael Gershon, *The Second Brain: A Groundbreaking New Understanding of Nervous Disorders of the Stomach and Intestine* (New York: HarperPerennial, 1999), preface.
3. www.mercola.com/2004/apr/14/splenda_reactions.htm.
4. Donna McCann, Angelina Barrett, Alison Cooper, et al., "Food Additives and Hyperactive Behaviour in 3-Year-Old and 8/9-Year-Old Children in the Community: A Randomised, Double-Blinded, Placebo-Controlled Trial," *The Lancet* 370 (2007): 1560–1567.
5. www.cspinet.org/reports/chemcuisine.htm.
6. Marion Nestle, *What to Eat* (New York: North Point Press, 2007), pp. 305–307.

Week 1: Nourish

1. www.sweetpoison.com/aspartame-sweeteners.html.
2. Nancy Appleton, *Lick the Sugar Habit* (New York: Avery, 1996), p. 68.

3. National Cancer Institute, "The Five a Day for Better Health Program," available at www.5aday.gov.

4. Centers for Disease Control and Prevention, "5 a Day Frequently Asked Questions: How Many Fruits and Vegetables Do Americans Eat?," available at www.cdc.gov/nccphp/dnpa/5ADay/faq/consumption_1.htm.

5. Walter Willett, "Trans Fats: The Story Behind the Label," *Harvard Public Health Review,* Spring 2006, available at www.hsph.harvard.edu/review/rvw_spring06/rvwspr06_transfats.html.

Week 2: Move

1. James Braly and Ron Hoggan, *Dangerous Grains* (New York: Avery, 2002), p. 3.

2. Ibid., p. 30.

3. T. Thompson, "Gluten Contamination of Commercial Oat Products in the United States," *The New England Journal of Medicine* 351 (2004): 2021–2022.

4. S. Storsrud et al., "Adult Coeliac Patients Do Tolerate Large Amounts of Oats," *European Journal of Clinical Nutrition* 57, no. 1 (2004): 163–169.

5. David Heber, *What Color Is Your Diet?* (New York: Regan Books, 2001), pp. 6–9.

6. C. F. Walker and B. E. Black, "Zinc and the Risk for Infectious Disease," *Annual Review of Nutrition* 24 (July 2004): 255–275.

7. Bruce W. Hollis, "Circulating 25-Hydroxyvitamin D Levels Indicative of Vitamin D Sufficiency: Implications for Establishing a New Effective Dietary Intake Recommendation for Vitamin D," *Journal of Nutrition* 135 (2005): 317–22.

8. P. Weber, "Vitamin E and Human Health: Rationale for Determining Recommended Intake Levels," *Nutrition* 13, no. 5 (1997): 450–460.

9. Anitra C. Carr and Balz Frei, "Toward a New Recommended Dietary Allowance for Vitamin C Based on Antioxidant and Health Effects in Humans," *The American Journal of Clinical Nutrition* 69, no. 6 (June 1999): 1086–1107.

10. National Research Council, *Recommended Dietary Allowances,* 10th ed. (Washington, D.C.: National Academy Press, 1989).

Week 3: Adapt

1. www.cholecalciferol-council.com.

2. Catherine M. Gordon, Kerrin C. DePeter, Henry A. Feldman, Estherann Grace, and S. Jean Emans, "Prevalence of Vitamin D Deficiency Among Healthy Adolescents," *Archives of Pediatric and Adolescent Medicine* 158 (2004): 531–537.

3. James P. Richardson, "Vitamin D Deficiency—The Once and Present Epidemic," editorial, *American Family Physician* (January 15, 2005): 24.

4. Michael F. Holick, "Vitamin D Deficiency: What a Pain It Is," editorial, *Mayo Clinic Proceedings* 78 (2003): 1457–1459.

Week 4: Release

1. "The Dangers of Soy," available at www.westonaprice.org.
2. David F. Brucker, "Effects of Environmental Synthetic Chemicals on Thyroid Function," *Thyroid* 8, no. 9 (1998): 827–856.
3. Viktor Gorlitzer von Mundy, "Influence of Fluorine and Iodine on the Metabolism, Particularly on the Thyroid Gland," *Muenchener Medicische Wochenschrift* 105 (1963): 182–186.
4. National Research Council, *Fluoride in Drinking Water: A Scientific Review of EPA's Standards* (Washington, D.C.: National Academies Press, 2006), pp. 197, 218, 222, 223.
5. www.fluoridealert.org/health/thyroid.
6. "Fluoridation is the greatest case of scientific fraud of this century," said by Robert Carlton, Ph.D., former U.S. EPA scientist, on *Marketplace,* Canadian Broadcast Company, November 24, 1992.
7. R. J. Carton and J. W. Hirzy, "Applying the NAEP Code of Ethics to the Environmental Protection Agency and the Fluoride in Drinking Water Standard," Proceedings of the 23rd Annual Conference of the National Association of Environmental Professionals, June 20–24, 1998.

Week 5: Balance

1. Available at www.forgivenessproject.com/stories/desmond=tutu.

Week 6: Sustain

1. Seventh amendment to the Cosmetics Directive, which came into force on March 1, 2005, published in *Official Journal of the European Union,* March 11, 2003.
2. Environmental Working Group's Cosmetic Database, available at www.cosmeticdatabase.com/research/whythismatters.php.
3. Ibid.
4. Ibid.
5. M. C. Kohn, F. Parham, S. A. Masten, C. J. Portier, M. D. Shelby, J. W. Brock, and L. L. Needham, "Human Exposure Estimates for Phthalates," *Environmental Health Perspectives* 108, no. 10 (October 2000): A440–A442.
6. Health Care Without Harm, "Aggregate exposure to phthalates in humans" (2002), available at www.noharm.org.
7. Sarah Graham, "Ubiquitous Chemical Associated with Abnormal Human Reproductive Development," *Scientific American,* May 27, 2005.
8. P. D. Darbre, A. Aljarrah, W. R. Miller, N. G. Coldham, M. J. Sauer, and G. S.

Pope, "Concentrations of Parabens in Human Breast Tumours," *Journal of Applied Toxicology* 24, no. 1 (January–February 2004): 5–13.

9. www.preventcancer.com/consumers/cosmetics/diethanolamine.html.

10. Roderick E. Black, Fred J. Hurley, and Donald C. Havery, "Occurrence of 1,4-Dioxane in Cosmetic Raw Materials and Finished Cosmetic Products," abstract, *Journal of AOAC International* 84, no. 3 (May 2001): 666–670.

11. U.S. Environmental Protection Agency, "1,4-Dioxane (1,4-Diethyleneoxide): Hazard Summary," created in April 1992, revised in January 2000, available at www.epa.gov/ttn/atw/hlthef/dioxane.html.

12. IARC Press Release, June 2004, available at www.iarc.fr/ENG/Press_Releases/archives/pr153a.html.

13. Health Canada, "Formaldehyde and Indoor Air," available at Health Canada's Web site, www.hc-sc.gc.ca/iyh-vsv/environ/formaldehyde_e.html.

14. "Formaldehyde," available at http://monographs.iarc.fr/ENG/Monographs/vol88/volume88.pdf.

15. B. L. Harlow, D. W. Cramer, D. A. Bell, and W. R. Welch, "Perineal Exposure to Talc and Ovarian Cancer Risk," *Obstetrics & Gynecology* 80 (1992): 19–26.

16. National Toxicology Program, "Toxicology and Carcinogenesis Studies of Talc (CAS no. 14807-96-6) (Non-Asbestiform) in F344/N Rats and B6C3F, Mice (Inhalation Studies)," Technical Report Series No. 421, National Toxicology Program, Washington, D.C.: Department of Health and Human Services, September 1993.

17. "Safety of Propylene Glycol," available at www.en.wikipedia.org/wiki/Propylene_glycol#Applications.

18. K. L. Rule, V. R. Ebbett, and P. J. Vikesland, "Formation of Chloroform and Chlorinated Organics by Free-Chlorine-Mediated Oxidation of Triclosan," *Environmental Science & Technology* 39, no. 9 (2005): 3176–3185.

19. Nik Veldhoen, Rachel C. Skirrow, Heather Osachoff, Heidi Wigmore, David J. Clapson, Mark P. Gunderson, Graham Van Aggelen, and Caren C. Helbing, "The Bactericidal Agent Triclosan Modulates Thyroid Hormone–Associated Gene Expression and Disrupts Postembryonic Anuran Development," *Aquatic Toxicology* 80, no. 3 (December 2006): 217–227.

20. "Plain Soap as Effective as Antibacterial but Without the Risk," available at www.physorg.com/news106418144.html.

21. M. N. Gadaleta, A. Cormio, V. Pesce, A. M. Lezza, and P. Cantatore, "Aging and Mitochondria," *Biochimie* 80, no. 10 (October 1998): 863–870.

22. R. T. Matthews, L. Yang, S. Browne, M. Baik, and M. F. Beal, "Coenzyme Q10 Administration Increases Brain Mitochondrial Concentrations and Exerts Neuroprotective Effects," *Proceedings of the National Academy of Sciences, USA* 95, no. 15 (July 21, 1998): 8892–8897.

23. T. M. Hagen, J. Liu, J. Lykkesfeldt, et al., "Feeding Acetyl-L-Carnitine and

Lipoic Acid to Old Rats Significantly Improves Metabolic Function While Decreasing Oxidative Stress," *Proceedings of the National Academy of Sciences USA* 99, no. 4 (February 19, 2002): 1870–1875.

24. H. Atamna, B. N. Ames, and J. Liu, "Delaying Aging with Mitochondrial Micronutrients and Antioxidants," *Scientific World Journal* 1, no. 1 (suppl. 3) (January 1, 2001): 81–82.

What to Do Now

1. Sidney MacDonald Baker with Karen Baar, *The Circadian Prescription: Get in Step with your Body's Natural Rhythms to Maximize Energy, Vitality, and Longevity* (New York: Putnam, 2000), pp. 22–25, 45–47.

2. www.newscientist.com/article/mg13217924.700-light-dawns-on-the-body-clock.

Troubleshooting

1. R. Bunevicius, A. J. Prange, et al., "T3 Helps with Hypothyroidism," *The New England Journal of Medicine* 340 (1999): 424–429, 469–470.

ACKNOWLEDGMENTS

Frank's Acknowledgments

To write a book takes a village. A heartfelt appreciation to the following special people whom I have been blessed to have in my life.

First, a big thank-you to my patients, for entrusting yourselves to my care. It is a great privilege to be your partner in health. *You* inspired *Spent*.

Thanks to my family. To Janice, my anchor, for loving, nurturing, supporting, and keeping me in rhythm and for sharing her delicious recipes. So much of this book and what I do would not be possible without you. To Ali, our beautiful daughter, for bringing so much joy into my life. Your comments and editing suggestions were so insightful. This book was truly a family creation. I love you both. And to Lily, Jeff, Marianne, Mikki, Cecil, David, and Michelle—our family, who gave us the roots to grow.

Thanks to my staff at the 1111 Wellness Center, particularly Vicky Zodo and Vanessa Echeveria, who keep my practice running in a steady rhythm so I can move to other beats.

A special thank-you to those who helped make this book a reality. To Mollie Doyle for your brilliance, patience, style, and love of the beat. Your understanding of the subject and ability to take a mass of information and create a user-friendly book continually astounds me. It has been such a gift to work with you. To Stephanie Tade for believing in me, having a vision, planting a seed, and overseeing its growth into *Spent*. To Lindsey Clennell for being such a wise and loving father, brother, mentor, colleague, and friend. Your yoga advice and wisdom are diffused throughout the book. To Kristi Anderson, Nathan Briner, and Yvonne De Kock, for imparting your knowledge and being such great models for the photographs. To Linda

Gaunt and Heidi Krupp, for your enthusiasm and eagerness to spread the word. To Beth Galton, for the exquisite yoga and exercise photos. To Timothy White, for my jacket photo and all your support.

Thanks to the people I call my Daily Advisory Committee—I call on you for so many things, and you always respond with wisdom, humor, and insight. To Fiona Druckenmiller, for everything you do in this world. To Donna Karan, for your enormous heart and commitment to changing the way patients are cared for. To Harriet Beinfield, Lic. Ac., and Efrem Korngold, O.M.D., Lic. Ac., for teaching me to see the world differently and supporting my growth ever since. To Larry Baskind, M.D., and Steven Cowan, M.D., rhythm brothers, for keeping me laughing and being there for the Lipman family whenever we needed you. To Jeff Bland, Ph.D., for fathering functional medicine and initiating a new, healthier direction in medicine. To Gabrielle Roth, queen of rhythm, for making me change my beat midcourse. To Alejandro Junger, M.D., for your charm, big heart, and love of life. To Kevin Law for saying it like it is and keeping my finger on the pulse. To Marcelle Pick, N.P., for your encouragement, love, and support. To Scott Berliner, R.Ph., for continually sharing your knowledge. To Bob Thurman, for your brilliance and willingness to impart your infinite wisdom. To Gil Chimes, D.C., acupuncturist and body worker extraordinaire, for keeping my body in tune. To Lori Benton, for giving me the title *Spent*. To Denis Crosley for your creative advice. And to Chris Blackwell, for your love of rhythm and turning the world on to such great music.

Thanks to all the folks at Touchstone Fireside: Trish Todd, for getting *Spent* from the get-go; Chris Lloreda, for getting 100 percent behind it; Zach Schisgal, for a great editing job; Shawna Lietzke, for being so helpful; publisher, Mark Gompertz, and director of publicity, Marcia Burch; Jessica Roth; and Lynn Anderson, for copyediting.

I am honored to be part of two amazing grassroots organizations working in the new South Africa, the Ubuntu Education Fund and MonkeyBiz. Thanks to Jacob Lief, Malizole "Banks" Gwaxula, Gcobani Zonke, Qondakele Sompondo, Mava Delpu, Jana Zindell, Jordan Levy, and all the staff and board of the Ubuntu Fund, and to Barbara Jackson and all the women at MonkeyBiz. You have brought so much more meaning into my life.

Thanks to all the friends and colleagues who have supported me over the years and with this book in particular: Patti Gift; Yves Durif; Paulette Cole; Kevin Bacon; Kyra Sedgwick; Richard Smith; Barry Schechter; Maria Hinojosa; Ronna Lichtenberg; Bobby Clennell; Susan Luck, RN; Charlene Chai; Barbara Locker; Marty Jaramillo, P.T.; Jill Pettijohn; Annie Jubb; Kate Horrigan, P.T.; Mark Hyman, M.D.; Woodson Merrell, M.D.; Robert Palmer, D.C.; Charlie DeFrancesco; Rob Di Stefano, D.C.; Lorraine Tiezzi; Susan Swimmer; Amy Homes; and Adam Banning.

Thanks to Rancho La Puerta and all the amazing staff for being my own personal Spent Solution.

To the Environmental Working Group (www.EWG.org) for the important work that they do.

Thanks to South Africa, for instilling in me African rhythms and Ubuntu.

Thanks to the pioneers in this new health movement, whose work has influenced me, in particular Christiane Northrup, M.D.; Mary Dunn; Annemarie Colbin, Ph.D., CHES; Annie Berthold Bond; Barbara Dossey, Ph.D., RN; Harriet Beinfield, Lic. Ac.; Efrem Korngold, O.M.D., Lic. Ac.; Jeff Bland, Ph.D.; Lindsey Clennell; Rodney Yee; Jim Gordon, M.D.; Larry Dossey, M.D.; Andrew Weil, M.D.; Alan Gaby, M.D.; Jonathan Wright, M.D.; Leo Galland, M.D.; Sidney Baker, M.D.; Jon Kabat-Zinn, Ph.D.; Richard Schaub, Ph.D.; Leon Chaitow, D.O., Alejandro Claraco, M.D.; Mark Seem, Ph.D.; Mark Blumenthal; Mike Adams.

To His Holiness the Dalai Lama, Nelson Mandela, Archbishop Desmond Tutu, and B. K. S. Iyengar, for shining their light on the path— thank you.

To Jon Stewart, Stephen Colbert, Bill Maher, and the late Richard Pryor and George Carlin, for keeping me laughing.

To all the musicians around the world who have kept me in rhythm with their music: Bob Marley, Bob Dylan, Michael Franti, Wyclef Jean, Manu Chao, Baaba Maal, Youssou N'Dour, Hugh Masakela, Abdullah Ibrahim, Angelique Kidjo, Gilberto Gil, Neil Young, Miles Davis, Van Morrison, Keith Jarrett, and Bill Laswell, to mention just a few.

Thank you all.

Janice's Acknowledgments

So many talented chefs, cooks, and friends have inspired me over the years. I am especially grateful to my mother, Mikki Norton, who taught me the pleasures of home cooking. Thanks to Mollie Katzen, Deborah Madison, Myrna Rosen, Annemarie Colbin, Martha Stewart, Jill Pettijohn, and Annie Jubb. Your recipes have guided and nourished us on this journey—a big thank-you. However, Frank and our incredible daughter, Alison, provide me with the greatest nourishment of all—their love. Special thanks to Lynne Kalvin, Felicity Schwartz, and Susan Cowan for their love and support. And finally, a very big thank-you to Mollie Doyle for helping me and making this process so smooth.

Mollie's Acknowledgments

Frank Lipman, for including me in this incredible project. I am honored and humbled.

Stephanie Tade, for her wisdom and humor.

Janice Lipman, for her delicious food and editorial intuition.

My husband, Thomas Bena, for going on the adventure.

INDEX

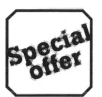

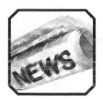

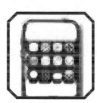

We hope you enjoyed this Hay House book.
If you would like to receive a free catalogue featuring additional
Hay House books and products, or if you would like information
about the Hay Foundation, please contact:

Hay House UK Ltd
292B Kensal Rd • London W10 5BE
Tel: (44) 20 8962 1230; Fax: (44) 20 8962 1239
www.hayhouse.co.uk

✻✻✻

Published and distributed in the United States of America by:
Hay House, Inc. • PO Box 5100 • Carlsbad, CA 92018-5100
Tel.: (1) 760 431 7695 or (1) 800 654 5126;
Fax: (1) 760 431 6948 or (1) 800 650 5115
www.hayhouse.com

Published and distributed in Australia by:
Hay House Australia Ltd • 18/36 Ralph St • Alexandria NSW 2015
Tel.: (61) 2 9669 4299; Fax: (61) 2 9669 4144
www.hayhouse.com.au

Published and distributed in the Republic of South Africa by:
Hay House SA (Pty) Ltd • PO Box 990 • Witkoppen 2068
Tel./Fax: (27) 11 467 8904 • www.hayhouse.co.za

Published and distributed in India by:
Hay House Publishers India • Muskaan Complex • Plot No.3
B-2 • Vasant Kunj • New Delhi – 110 070.
Tel.: (91) 11 41761620; Fax: (91) 11 41761630.
www.hayhouse.co.in

Distributed in Canada by:
Raincoast • 9050 Shaughnessy St • Vancouver, BC V6P 6E5
Tel.: (1) 604 323 7100; Fax: (1) 604 323 2600

✻✻✻

Sign up via the Hay House UK website to receive the Hay House
online newsletter and stay informed about what's going on with
your favourite authors. You'll receive bimonthly announcements
about discounts and offers, special events, product highlights,
free excerpts, giveaways, and more!
www.hayhouse.co.uk